SH 7-4.

For Martha Bruner
With warmest best wishes

Signed

1200
97BB

PSYCHIATRY
IN THE
COMMUNIST
WORLD

PSYCHIATRY
IN THE
COMMUNIST
WORLD

Edited by ARI KIEV, M.D.

HEAD, CORNELL PROGRAM
IN SOCIAL PSYCHIATRY,
CORNELL MEDICAL COLLEGE,
NEW YORK HOSPITAL, NEW YORK CITY

SCIENCE HOUSE, New York

Contributors

Dr. Gregorio Bermann
Professor of Psychiatry
University of Cordoba
9 de julio 408
Cordoba
ARGENTINA

Dr. A. Dosies
Medical Chief of Psychiatric Service
University of Bucharest
Str. Macet 8 R.
Bucharest
RUMANIA

Dr. A. G. Galach'yan
Senior Scientific Worker
Institute of Psychiatry
Zagordnoe Chausse, D. 2
Moscow
U.S.S.R.

Dr. Tadeusz Gnat
Chief
Section on Psychiatry
Ministry of Health
Warsaw
POLAND

Dr. Stanislav Grof
Research Psychiatrist
Department of Psychiatry, Postgrad-
  uate
Medical Institute
Prague 8
CZECHOSLAVAKIA

Dr. Vladimir Jakovljevic
Docent of Faculty of Philosophy
Belgrade, studentski trgl
YUGOSLAVIA

Dr. D. Müller-Hegemann
Director
State Hospital for Psychiatry and
  Neurology
114 Berlin-Biesdorf
GERMANY

Dr. Julius Nyirö*
Professor of Psychiatry
Director, Psychiatric Clinic
University of Budapest
Budapest
HUNGARY

Dr. C. Parhon-Stefanescu
University of Bucharest
Str. Macet 8 R.
Bucharest
RUMANIA

Dr. V. Predescu
Senior Scientific Worker
University of Bucharest
Str. Macet 8 R.
Bucharest
RUMANIA

Dr. Joseph Prokupek
Associate Professor of Psychiatry
Head, Department of Psychiatry,
  Postgraduate
Medical Institute
Prague 8
CZECHOSLOVAKIA

Dr. Iordan Stoimenov
Senior Assistant
Department of Psychiatry
Higher Institute of Medicine
Sofia
BULGARIA

Dr. Jaroslav Stuchlik†
Emeritus Professor
University of Prague
Praha 2 Legerova 8, CSSR
Prague
CZECHOSLOVAKIA

Dr. Ivan Temkov
Professor of Psychiatry
Department of Psychiatry
Higher Institute of Medicine
Sofia
BULGARIA

* Died June, 1966
† Died 1967

Preface

IN THE PAST DECADE a number of psychiatrists have reported on psychiatry in the Soviet Union, Czechoslovakia, and Yugoslavia. These reports have been valuable in stimulating interest in the psychiatric theories and practices in these countries, especially those of the Soviet Union, which has been most visited. The present volume brings together for the first time material on most of the Communist countries, written by psychiatrists selected for their familiarity with the overall picture in the countries where they work. In some instances the psychiatrists were recommended by the Ministry of Health or by a professional medical association in their countries. Although letters to China and Albania were not answered, a contribution was received from Professor Gregorio Bermann of Cordoba University, Cordoba, Argentina, who has visited China several times.

An earlier volume, *Magic, Faith and Healing: Studies in Primitive Psychiatry Today*,* focused on the *wissenssoziologie* of psychiatry in pre-industrial and developing societies—that is, the interrelationships between their psychiatric systems and the social-historical contexts in which these

* Ari Kiev (ed.), Free Press of Glencoe, New York, 1964.

systems evolved. It was with the same general intention that the present volume on the Communist countries was conceived. Thus, we hoped to examine the significance of Marxist-Leninist ideology in relation to psychiatric theory and practice. However, these complex and highly diverse societies in Communist lands do not lend themselves to the type of analysis applied to the simpler societies. Although united by a common ideology, the Communist countries have generally dissimilar historical and cultural traditions, are in different stages of social and economic development, and pursue different national interests. Moreover, influences from other countries, as well as scientific developments, have created further differences between these countries and within each one. Hence, it seemed difficult to view them together and to clarify the relationships between various medical and psychiatric traditions and institutions which were often different even within a single country.

A recent trip to Poland, the Soviet Union, Bulgaria, Hungary, and Czechoslovakia confirmed this impression and increased my awareness of their wide range of approaches to psychiatry—a range indicated by the papers in this volume.

It should be emphasized that although contributors were asked to follow a general outline in their papers, they were allowed considerable leeway. Though their focus was to be comprehensive, their own biases and preferences have undoubtedly influenced the emphasis they have given to various aspects of psychiatry in their respective countries. All are busy, productive people whose views will inevitably reflect the type of activities in which they themselves are engaged. Hence, the papers should be viewed as preliminary characterizations of psychiatry in the Communist countries.

In addition to the contributors who made this volume possible, I am especially indebted to my wife, Phyllis Eve Kiev, who read various portions of the manuscript and provided the much-needed encouragement to pursue this project. I am grateful to Seymour Weingarten for his valuable editorial assistance during the final months of preparation. The cost of several translations was supported by a National Institute of Mental Health Program Project Grant held by Dr. Ernest M. Gruenberg, of Columbia University's College of Physicians and Surgeons, where I worked while preparing a major portion of this volume. I am grateful to him and to the National Institute of Mental Health. I am most appreciative of the generous advice given by Drs. A. B. Sneznevsky, Nikola Schipkowensky, Karl Leonhard, Andrzej Jus, and Mil Filipovic, who put me in touch with a number of the contributors.

ARI KIEV

Contents

CHAPTER ONE

Introduction

DR. ARI KIEV

PSYCHIATRY IS in principle concerned with the discovery and diagnosis, treatment and prevention of psychiatric disorders. In practice, however, these steps are sometimes circumvented and rarely, if ever, achieved. Unlike a disease such as tuberculosis, all cases of mental disorder can never be ascertained. Some individuals are not thought to be suffering from treatable conditions; others may suffer silently or impose their burdens on willing relatives. Furthermore, notions as to what factors constitute a case usually vary not only among laymen but among professionals as well. When a case is found, diagnostic methods and concepts generally vary. Indeed, if one is ever to be able to compare the incidence and prevalence of specific disorders over time and in different places, it will be necessary to obtain a consensus on the classification of psychiatric disorders and their nosology, just as it will be necessary to develop standardized instruments to identify cases and measure degrees of impairment. Such a consensus is particularly difficult to obtain because of the marked shortage of personnel in some countries; since psychiatrists find themselves with little free time from their service commitments, they are unable to fully investigate these matters.

Another contributing element may be that a variety of treatment methods have evolved, without sufficient understanding of why they are effective. This uncertainty lends itself to much speculation and has given rise to a variety of theories regarding the etiology of psychiatric disorders. For the same reasons, psychiatry has been more influenced by national and cultural patterns than by specific and necessary schemata. Indeed, unlike more defined and circumscribed sciences and technologies, psychiatry reflects the *Weltanschanung* and political, social, and philosophical premises of a society. Thus psychiatrists, using different methods and approaches in different social and cultural contexts, are concerned with different problems and have developed different emphases.

To progress as a scientific discipline, psychiatry requires greater uniformity in both its methods and its concepts. Such uniformity, in turn, demands that much be learned about the nature of psychiatric theory and practice in different parts of the world.

Examination of psychiatry in the Soviet Union, Eastern European countries, and China is of special value, in view of the explicit connection of psychiatry with the basic ideological premises of these societies. Indeed, the political and social ideology which these countries share is to a large extent concerned with planning social and medical services and the centralization of authority in administering these services.

Comparative studies of psychiatry are of interest in and of themselves and they also provide a broader perspective from which more uniform methods and concepts can evolve. It is for these purposes that the present volume has been prepared.

THE COMMUNIST COUNTRIES

Prior to World War II, social systems differed among what are now the Communist countries. Hungary, Poland, and Rumania had a large class of feudal aristocrats, but Bulgaria and Yugoslavia had none. Only Czechoslovakia contained a large group of industrialists; peasantry predominated everywhere else. There were large numbers of gypsies in several East European countries and thousands of pastoral peoples in Yugoslavia, Bulgaria, Greece, and Albania. In Albania and Montenegro large parts of the population were still existing on the tribal level, and in all of the societies there were large minority groups. The working class, beginning to develop, was powerful only in Czechoslovakia, where the Social Democratic and Communist parties were in existence. Similarly, the *petit bour-*

geoisie, although growing in most of the countries, was influential only in Czechoslovakia.

Peasants constituted 50 to 80 percent of the population in all the countries except Czechoslovakia, where they comprised only 34 percent. Agriculture in Poland, Austria, Hungary, and the old kingdom of Rumania was based largely on the landed estates, although in the Balkans small holdings prevailed. Some two-thirds to three-quarters of the peasants of Eastern Europe were small holders whose land was felt to be insufficient to support their families, partly because the level of industrialization was low and the methods of agriculture were backward.

After World War II, efforts were made to model these societies after the Soviet Union with special emphasis on collectivization and rapid industrialization. The policy in most of the societies was to strengthen the peasants both economically and socially through land reforms and nationalization of industry. The land reform in Eastern Europe consisted not only of acquiring what had been German property, but also of redistributing large land areas. At first the large landed estates were divided up and distributed among the peasantry. In time this policy was altered to allow the government to organize a more systematic method of exchange between rural and urban areas. Thus, agricultural development regulated by a central planning board proceeded into total collectivization.

By 1949 the first collective farms had appeared, varying with respect to possession of implements and land, work obligations, and the distribution of profits. Labor was to be paid according to state standards. Production quotas and produce delivery schedules were also established in accordance with state plans. In most regimes agricultural policy followed that of the Soviet Union. The state-centralized system of exchange between towns and villages involved quotas for deliveries of crops, changes in taxation, and the establishment of state-owned cooperative shops in the countryside. Efforts were also made to mechanize agriculture. The final stage of agricultural change was the elimination of the *kulaks* and establishment of collectivization.

Industrialization and the collectivization of agriculture proceeded more rapidly in China than elsewhere. Prior to 1949 over 80 percent of the population, the majority peasants, lived in rural areas. With industrialization in one generation as its major goal, the state made efforts to develop rural industry, utilize manpower fully, and mechanize agriculture. First land was redistributed to the peasants, then agricultural cooperatives were established, and finally, in 1956, communes were established. At the same time, the state assumed increasing control over private enterprise, the labor market, the allocation of raw materials, and sales and marketing. By 1956 all major industries had been socialized.

At present, agriculture is fully or partly collectivized in China, East Germany, Czechoslovakia, Bulgaria, and Rumania. In Yugoslavia and Poland it remains essentially privately operated. In 1961, 98 percent of the farms in Bulgaria, 86.7 percent of those in Czechoslovakia, 85.3 percent of those in Rumania, and 87.2 percent in Hungary were collectivized. The process of collectivizing lands increased surplus manpower, so that more people could move to the cities and work in new industries. The shifts of population from rural to urban areas were especially marked in Yugoslavia, China, and Poland, which changed from predominantly agricultural so-cieties to mixed industrial-agricultural types. Countries such as Hungary, with the most inequitable prewar distribution of land, underwent the greatest agrarian transformations. The more industrialized of the countries —Czechoslovakia, for example—suffered the least economic dislocation. With changes in the agricultural sphere, large-scale industrialization was encouraged to enable the surplus argicultural population to be absorbed into urban areas and to provide a market for agricultural products. These programs to expand heavy industry were modeled on the Five-Year Plan of the Soviet Union.

By 1948, industry, banking, and wholesale trade were all nationalized. In 1949, to bring economic aid to the Eastern European countries, the Soviet Union created the Council for Mutual Economic Aid. By 1951, there was increased commerce between the Soviet Union and the other Eastern European countries, particularly East Germany, Poland, Hungary, and Czechoslovakia. Most of these nations relied heavily on the Soviet Union for capital and equipment for their own industrialization. About 80 percent of the trade of the Eastern European countries is with other Com-munist countries, although this has been changing in recent years. As the major source of raw materials, industrial equipment, and technological know-how and as a major market, the Soviet Union accounts for one-third to one-half of the foreign trade of most Eastern European countries.

Although there have been shifts in the specific emphases given to heavy versus light industry from time to time, it is fair to say that the pre-dominant trend in the Communist countries, especially in East Germany, Russia, and Czechoslovakia, has been the progressive development of in-dustrialization. In 1913, two percent of the persons in the Soviet Union were factory workers. In 1926, twenty percent of the workers were engaged in industrial occupations, and by 1939, twenty-five million peasants had migrated from rural collectives to urban areas to become part of the urban labor force. Similarly, in China the first Five-Year Plan before the Great Leap Forward (1958–1961) allocated 41 percent of the investment into industry and 19 percent into agriculture. The emphasis on reconstruction, industrialization, and the mechanization of agriculture has been associated with attempts to solve the problem of surplus agricultural workers, migration, and urbanization. Moreover, the rapid pace of industrialization has been linked to the problems of food shortage and refugees as well as to various social and political issues well known to the student of current events.

ORGANIZATION OF HEALTH SERVICES

With every regime's emphasis on manpower to rapidly build a modern industrialized society, the individual's health and morale, as key assets to the system, became a major concern of the state. After World War II, the practice of psychiatry became part of the health services available throughout the Communist world. In fact, all health institutions, pharmacies, and the organizations supervising the production and distribution of supplies were nationalized. The aim was to provide increased free care to broader segments of the population. Administration of medical institutions was allocated to the Ministry of Public Health and Social Welfare in each country. Five-year reconstruction plans to increase the number of doctors and hospital beds and to expand facilities were undertaken.

Though varying from country to country, facilities have in general been expanding since the war. In Rumania there were 4,211 psychiatric beds in 1938; now there are 12,000. In 1937 Czechoslovakia had 16,909 psychiatric beds, representing more than 23 percent of all hospital beds, or 1.17 psychiatric beds per 1,000 inhabitants. By the end of 1963, there were 18,683 psychiatric beds, some 10.9 percent of all hospital beds, or 1.36 per 1,000 inhabitants. The figures Jakovlejic cites for Yugoslavia provide an interesting contrast. In 1945, there were 0.19 psychiatric beds per 1,000 inhabitants: in 1950, 0.45 beds; and in 1963, 0.67 beds. This ratio falls below the minimum of 1 bed per 1,000 inhabitants (which is recommended by the World Health Organization). The 12,691 psychiatric beds in Yugoslavia constitute only 12.1 percent of the total number of patient beds in that country. Counting the beds in special institutions as well as in mental hospitals, Bulgaria has 6,477 beds, or 0.81 per 1,000 population—

also below standard. However, active construction has proceeded, and by 1980, a figure of 1.5 per 1,000 is expected. In 1949, there were only 90,000 hospital beds in all of China for a population of close to 500 million, including between 100 and 6,000 psychiatric beds (the figures cited by two different reports in 1949 and 1948 respectively), and not more than 60 psychiatrists. In 1959, on the tenth anniversary of the Revolution, 62 new psychiatric hospitals, with a number of beds 14 times greater than before, were reported to have been built.

Social security and sickness-insurance schemes have also been expanded. Although Eastern European countries have long had social security in the form of compulsory social insurance, particularly for old-age disability and illness, after the war the range of benefits and the number of occupations and individuals covered was increased in most of these countries.

National insurance legislation implemented the economic and social policies of the various governments and favored the socialized sector over the private sector, industry over agriculture, heavy over light industry, and higher types of agriculture cooperatives over lower types. For example, in some countries health insurance did not extend to private entrepreneurs, private farmers, or farmers in the lower types of agricultural cooperatives. Medical care was to a large extent determined by the direction which the economy had taken. Thus, large industrial establishments were equipped with infirmaries, consultation-and-treatment centers, polyclinics, etc. The legal right to social insurance was a privilege effectively afforded only to active builders of socialism who fulfilled their responsibilities, plans, and tasks, and maintained political and trade-union discipline.

During maternity leave, a worker received special wage compensation, as well as special compensation for motherhood. Special awards were given to mothers who bore many children. That this approach was linked to the needs of the society was indicated by the fact that women were encouraged to return to work as soon as possible and that most plants provided nurseries and kindergartens for children of working mothers.

Social security and medical benefits were based on Lenin's notions that "he who does not work shall not eat," and that "the administration of social insurance should be meted out to each according to his work." Thus, the social-security system was integrally related to state goals, especially to the interests of production. Social-security benefits were sometimes dependent on membership in trade unions, length of employment in a given enterprise, the kind and place of work, and the extent of adherence to socialized-labor discipline. Benefits under social security were comparable to benefits elsewhere. Persons with fascist backgrounds or with views inimicable to the state were excluded from benefits. In some places, trade-union members received full benefits, while nonmembers received only 50 percent of the established rate. People who were privately employed, or self-employed, had to pay higher premiums.

Health protection in Eastern Europe was thus made a system of governmental, community, or collective measures which had as their aims the prevention and treatment of illness, the provision of healthy working and living conditions, and a high work capacity, as well as a higher life expectancy for the individual. Health measures, part of the respective regimes' overall plans for industrialization and collectivization of agriculture, allowed theoretically for rational allocation of personnel, funds, and other scarce resources, organization of medical facilities, and provision of services with maximum efficiency.

Supervision of most activities was concentrated into a central organization, the Health Ministry, which directed, coordinated, and standardized medical and public health efforts. Branches were set up at all major administrative territorial divisions of the various countries. The costs of medical services were underwritten by the state and financed through general revenues and taxation. The direction of medicine began, then, with the central government and extended to each territorial administrative level. Thus, in every Communist country there was a rather elaborate hierarchy.

The range of psychiatric treatment facilities that has been developed throughout Eastern Europe is extensive. Besides traditional mental hospitals and outpatient clinics, there are special institutions for the treatment of oligophrenics, epileptics, and alcoholics. In recent years units of 25 to 100 beds for the treatment of milder psychiatric disorders have been opened in general hospitals, and attempts are being made to end the separation of somatic from mental cases. Child-guidance clinics, municipal child-welfare committees, and schools, as well as special institutions for antisocial personalities, have been established. There are, in addition, a number of special programs in some of the Communist countries. In the Czech spas of Karlsbad, Marienbad, Piestany, and Jesenik, patients recovering from all degrees of psychiatric illness can receive mineral-water treatment. In Poland, where rehabilitation measures have been extensively developed, there is cottage industry for the handicapped who cannot come to the sheltered or cooperative establishments and family-care programs in the agricultural regions.

Hospitals care for the acutely ill, and chronically ill patients are often referred to chronic colonies: however, the major emphasis is on community-centered outpatient treatment, with continuity of care for all phases of psychiatric illness. Efforts are made to maintain an active statistical count of patients who come under the care of the clinic. Such registers, which record every type of treatment the patient receives, are also helpful in surveys of patients who need psychiatric treatment or supportive care. In many clinics one finds units for social therapy, rehabilitation, vocational guidance, and industrial training, as well as sheltered workshops.

Rehabilitation of chronic mental patients is one of the more actively developed disciplines in the Communist countries. Graduated programs from simple occupational therapy to sheltered agricultural and factory workshops provide opportunity at all stages of treatment for patients to obtain some degree of social remission, even when the clinical prognosis is guarded. In Poland, as Gnat points out, the type of job available depends partly on regional manpower needs and partly on the possibilities of employment in the shared-work establishments (cooperatives) for the handicapped and in industry. Psychiatric clinics also maintain contacts with municipal public-assistance boards and provide financial, housekeeping, and nursing help for psychiatric patients living at home.

Clinics provide comprehensive psychiatric treatment for all kinds of patients, except those in need of hospitalization. They also provide vocational, financial, legal, and educational support when indicated. Public health preventive measures are provided through educational talks to clinics, factories, and various organizations. Attempts are also made to visit patients in their own homes, with a view toward patients being treated entirely at home or as outpatients in the outpatient clinic. In 1964 in Bulgaria, 196,484 ambulatory patients were seen, of which 22,424, or 11.5 percent, were examined in their homes. Suitable patients are examined or specially treated in active day hospitals and treatment centers; thus, the doctor sustains contact with the patient. By remaining with his family, the patient can maintain his security and continue to live in the community instead of becoming an enforced member of a group in a mental hospital (an artificial environment which bears little resemblance to ordinary home life). With such a program custodial and chronic hospital patterns are less likely to develop and the number of chronic, hospitalized patients is kept down.

In less developed areas, the priority given to psychiatric disorders ranks low. This is particularly true of countries such as Albania, where mortality is high on account of infectious diseases, malaria, tuberculosis, sleeping sickness, yellow fever, yaws, amoebic dysentery, nutritional-deficiency diseases, and intestinal parasitism. Underdeveloped areas in Eastern Europe have few qualified psychiatrists and few facilities for training more. Treatment facilities are frequently so scarce that it is necessary to travel several hundred miles to a central mental hospital. Hence patients, when admitted, are often in the latter stages of illness. There are too few general hospitals with adequate psychiatric facilities, and those mental hospitals which exist are overcrowded.

PSYCHIATRIC THEORY

The history of psychiatry in the Communist world—an important factor in a consideration of its psychiatric theory—differs widely among the countries, particularly in the extent of their traditions of modern psychiatry. Whereas in Czechoslovakia the first autonomous asylum for patients was established in 1458, in Znojmo, Moravia, modern psychiatric facilities were not introduced until 1844, in the "New House" of the Prague Hospital. Here the most modern methods, especially rehabilitative measures, were employed. In Poland psychiatric care probably began in the sixteenth century with the establishment of *hospitale delirantium*. Developments here paralleled those in Western Europe, and a firm classical tradition was established by the nineteenth century. The first insane asylum in Hungary was established in 1840, from which time can be dated the beginning of scientific psychiatry in that country.

Similarly, in Rumania, modern psychiatric care was not initiated until the early nineteenth century. Prior to that time, care of mental patients had been a function of the monasteries—a pattern common throughout Eastern Europe. It should be noted, though, as Parhon-Stefanescu does in the chapter on Rumania, that medical considerations regarding the mentally ill did exist in this earlier period. In the legal code of Volvade of Valachie, written in 1652, the role of the doctor in assessing insanity is emphasized, as is the notion that insane persons should be cared for instead of being punished for crimes they commit. In 1838, the care of the insane became the responsibility of the government. Work therapy was first applied in Rumania in 1859, at the monastery in Marcutya, under the supervision of a physician, Dr. Protici. By 1897, a chair of psychiatry was established at the monastery.

In Russia, the first special institution for the insane was established in

1762 at a "special home" in Novgorod. Under the czars, psychiatric services were well organized in the regions and cities. Of special significance was the scientific tradition initiated by workers such as Korsakov and Kandinsky at the end of the nineteenth century.

The progress of psychiatry in Yugoslavia reflects, in part, the stages at which various areas were developed. To this day, exorcism is practiced in the Balkans, charms are used in Macedonia, and folk medicine is popular in the East, although the western regions had more contact with Western Europe. In 1804, the first department for the mentally ill in a public hospital was established in Zagreb. By 1856, humane legislation had been passed, and in 1861, the first hospital for mental disease was built in Belgrade.

Developments were slower in Bulgaria, where the Turkish yoke retarded progress until the nineteenth century. Bulgaria's first psychiatric department was not established until 1888 at the Aleksandrovska Hospital in Sofia. As elsewhere in Eastern Europe, the predominant influences were at first German, but soon came to be Russian. Especially significant was the work of the Russian N. M. Popov, who introduced the first textbook of psychiatry into Bulgaria.

China's history of psychiatry goes back to the fourteenth century B.C. Writings from that century already indicated an awareness of psychiatric illness. In the year 1060 A.D. at the Imperial College of Medicine, 30 out of 100 students studied "illness of the wind." In the year 1608, during the Ming dynasty, Wang K'en-tang divided psychiatric illnesses into three groups: alienation, madness, and fits. In 1610 A.D. Ch'ao Iluang-fang described fifty-nine nervous mental diseases. The first modern psychiatric institution, a hospital with thirty beds, was introduced in Canton in 1897 by Dr. John Kerr, an American. During the twentieth century, numerous small missionary hospitals were established throughout the country, and courses in psychiatry were introduced into the medical-school curriculum. Chinese psychiatry has been progressively influenced by German, American, and Russian psychiatry, and more recently by the resurgence of traditional Chinese medicine with its emphasis on cauterization, acupuncture, and herbal remedies. In 1965, some 350,000 practitioners and eighteen of the ninety medical schools were dedicated to this traditional approach.

Contemporary events tend to make us forget that in the past many of the Communist countries had strong ties with the West. The first director of the Health Service in Rumania, Dr. Carol Davila, had been trained in France, where he became familiar with the ideas of Pinel. Professor

Alexandre Obregia, the second professor of psychiatry in Bucharest, had worked in the laboratories of Virchow, Munk, and Westphal in Germany, and in French clinics with Charcot, Magnan, and Ball.

In Yugoslavia the influence of the western European countries, especially France, was reflected in the introduction of modern diagnostic and treatment methods in 1881 by Jovan Danic, who had worked in Paris. Of interest, too, is the fact that in 1920, the professor in Ljubljana was Alfred Serko, a disciple of Wagner-Jauregg and a student of both Freud and Adler.

During the late nineteenth century, when a search for organic factors dominated European psychiatry, the predominant theories in Eastern European countries were based on the notion of diseases of the brain. The names of Kuffner in Czechoslovakia, Korsakov in Russia, Krustnikov in Bulgaria, Sechenov, Gannushkin, and Gilyarovsky in Russia, and Jan Mazurkiewicz in Poland, deserve special mention. In Czechoslovakia, F. Kostel introduced fever therapy by means of the inoculation of artificial variola in cases of general paresis. In the early years of this century, Professor Constantine Parhon introduced the study of endocrine disorders as etiological factors in mental illness—an area still of considerable interest.

Developments in Western Europe were felt to a considerable extent in all but the Balkan states and the Soviet Union. While the history of psychiatry differed from country to country, all seem to have shared the continental emphasis on an organic approach to mental disorders, a trend which persists to the present. Of the various organic conceptions of psychiatry, Pavlov's seems to have become the conception most accepted in recent years. Indeed, the tie-in of political and social theory with the views of Pavlov is one of the most striking features of psychiatric theorizing in several Communist countries, particularly the Soviet Union. Notably, a central concept of dialectical materialism views the individual as subordinate to the group and its goals and cites social changes as bringing about changes in personality. This finds support in Pavlov's notion of personality development, which, like Communist theory, stresses rational factors and the importance of social change.

In the Communist countries, mental phenomena are considered secondary to material processes, and psychological life is seen as unfolding within the context of a larger social life. This view does not seek to explain social movements and social conditions in terms of individual psychology and does not emphasize childhood experiences as crucial for the genesis of personality and psychological disorders. Experiences beyond childhood are considered equally crucial in determining the individual's psychology. Pavlov's theory supported the notion that men could be conditioned by appropriate first- and second-order stimuli—that is, an appropriately controlled environment—to achieve almost any kind of social adaption. A Communist environment is believed to be the one which best develops proper moral-psychological characteristics and, then, prevents neuroses due to nonadaptive cortical reflexes.

In psychopathology Pavlov distinguished two symptom groups in disease: those conditioned directly by damaging factors such as infection, trauma, or tumor, which produce primary symptoms, and those arising indirectly, or secondarily to the pathological focus, as defensive measures. Primary symptoms were to be treated by detoxification and neutralization, while secondary symptoms were to be supported and intensified. Thus, symptoms of psychoses and neuroses were viewed as conditioned reflexes developed through environmental influences. If noxious environmental factors were eliminated, the disease phenomena would be extinguished regardless of primary symptoms.

It should be emphasized that Pavlovian theory, supporting the general Communist emphasis on the role of social factors, has in turn received official support from the Soviet government, which has thus strengthened its central role in Soviet psychiatry. The acceptance of Pavlovian theory is accompanied by a rejection of those theories which regard unconscious thoughts as motivating forces over which man has little control. Such theories are obviously incompatible with a system which sets great store in rational planning for society and for the individual. Moreover, "dynamic" theories are seen as having limited social usefulness, since they deny the notion of man's perfectability and ignore the importance of the social environment.

Psychoanalysis and the kind of unconscious determinism it represents is rejected also because of its suggestive, arbitrary character. Inasmuch as it fails to utilize generally accepted methods for substantiating scientific data, it is seen as distracting attention from the real potential of public health medicine and prophylaxis. Psychoanalysis is rejected on the further grounds that Freudian theory exaggerated the role of sexual instincts, schematized the analysis of neurotic genetic factors, and oversimplified the interpretation of the patient's introspection. Since the thirties most European psychiatrists have been critical of the Freudian psychoanalytic focus on understanding the *meaning* of symptoms rather than the *mechanism* of symptom formation. Whereas a Pavlovian approach to neurotic disorders tends to focus on how people develop specific kinds of symptoms, the Freudian system emphasizes the significance of symptoms in terms of psychopathological background, or pathogenesis.

Although Pavlovian theory is predominant in the Soviet Union, Poland, Bulgaria, and Czechoslovakia, other European influences have also been important. We find a good example of this in the writings of Nikola Schipkowensky, a professor of psychiatry in Sofia, Bulgaria. His well-known monograph, *Pathologische Realisationen der Personlichlkeit* (Pathological Reactions of Personality) Vol. 1,* which combined Pavlovian and Kraepelinian theories with dynamic interpretations of social, biological, and personality factors, suggests a nosologic system based on the concept of specific disease entities. He clearly diffentiates psychiatric reactions from illness. Reactions imply a definite cause-and-effect relationship between an event and a psychological condition and the possibility of cure through psychotherapy using the patient's subjective experience of the cause.

For Schipkowensky, hysteria is a disease entity which in Pavlovian terms can be said to result from psychic trauma threatening the life or the highest values of a person, who reacts according to his particular constitution. Thus, where emotions supersede reason, the individual is most susceptible. This trauma provokes a "reversion of bodily activity," so that digestion becomes vomiting and circulation is channeled to the skin.

At the end of the war, V. Vujic's (Belgrade) theory of larval encephalitis and similar notions of central-nervous-system inflammation or intoxications were in Yugoslavia the principal explanations of neurotic symptomatology. Since then, various admixtures of dynamic theory, reflexogical theory, and the constitutional approach have been combined in a most active eclecticism. The influence of Fromm and Horney is especially evident at the Dr. D. Misovic Hospital in Belgrade, while the theories of Kretschmer and Schultz are emphasized in Ljubljana.

In Hungary, Professor Gyula Nyirö, who died in June, 1966, was the dominant figure in psychiatry. He regarded the nervous system as a complex organization of chemodynamics and this provided the theoretical foundation for his explanation of response formation and extinction. He believed that basic to man's psychic activities is the differentiation between object and self. Working with conditioned reflexes he maintained that the lower-level stereotypes display collective characteristics which become typical of certain communities, families, or even nationalities.

---

* Vienna, 1960 (210 pp.).

THE INCIDENCE AND PREVALENCE OF PSYCHIATRIC DISORDERS

It is generally accepted that the incidence of psychosis does not vary greatly from one country to another. The World Health Organization in 1958 estimated the rate of psychosis between 3 and 7 per 1,000 population. Increased rates of neurosis have been reported throughout the world, particularly in westernizing or industrializing areas, but these data are not well established.

Incidence and prevalence rates of mental disorders, ordinarily difficult to ascertain, are even more difficult to establish and assess for comparative purposes.

The very different patterns described in the chapters on Yugoslavia, Bulgaria, and China emphasize the difficulty in generalizing about such rates. It should be noted, too, that differences between Eastern European and Western psychiatrists' orientations toward diagnostic entities appear to affect rate differences. For example, Eastern European psychiatrists are in general critical of Kretschmer's notion that quirks of the normal personality can develop into psychoses—the kind of view which Galach'yan considers to have led "to an unjustified view of schizophrenia with . . . severe consequences for persons thus classified as mentally ill." Among Eastern European psychiatrists an effort is made to distinguish between neurotic and psychotic disorders, whereas in the West the tendency is to view mental illness as a continuum.

In some Communist countries the overall incidence of mental disorder is asserted to be lower than in the Western World. This lower incidence is attributed to the people's unity in the common purpose of building up Communist societies, to the slower tempo of life, to the fact that individuals have fewer decisions to make, and to a group life which involves the mental and emotional therapy of sharing one another's problems and affairs.

We should note, however, that Nyirö reports a 23 percent increase in patients discharged from mental and neurological institutions in Hungary in the last five years. Similarly Jakovljevic reports an increase in various psychiatric disorders in Yugoslavia. In fact, his data point to a progressive increase in the number of cases and the rate of psychiatric morbidity from 1950 to 1962. In 1962 the number of cases was eleven times as great as that in 1950, and the rate per 1,000 population was nine times as great.

Inasmuch as many parts of Yugoslavia have not developed adequate facilities, the true prevalence of psychiatric morbidity is probably even higher. It is still difficult to accurately assess historical trends regarding rates since much of the increase can be attributed to increasingly tolerant attitudes toward mental illness among general practitioners, psychiatrists, and the public. An increase in the prevalence of psychiatric morbidity is also reported for Bulgaria: in 1952 the rate was 0.73; by 1964 it had increased to 9.94. It is difficult to determine, though, whether this higher rate reflects an increased incidence of psychiatric disorder or merely the increased availability of clinics and other facilities. There can be little doubt that increased use of psychiatric facilities accounts for at least part of the increase, since a greater number of patients are admitted to clinics in their first month of illness. In 1962, 7.2 percent of all Bulgarian psychiatric patients had been admitted to clinics in the first month of illness. By 1964 the rate was 12.4 percent in the country as a whole and 17.2 percent in Sofia.

Because rates of incidence of the major psychoses, such as schizophrenia, are approximately the same in capitalist and Communist countries, differences in total rates reflect differences in frequency of the less severe psychiatric disorders, such as the neuroses. In Communist nations, as in the West, schizophrenia is regarded as the major psychiatric disorder. Major psychoses are said to be biologically caused and to be related to the social environment. Minor psychogenic disorders, on the other hand, are thought to be caused by environmental stresses, and the smaller number of these cases and their continuing diminution are explained by the notion that conflict between the exploiting and the exploited classes has been dissolved and classes have been abolished. Thus, homosexuality and other sexual deviations reported absent in most Communist countries are associated with capitalist morals. In Czechoslovakia, where such conditions are said to exist, they are attributed to residual capitalist influences; in other words, deviant individuals are not proper members of the new society.

Other factors said to contribute to the lower incidence of psychiatric disorder are the greater number of women working, the abolition of private property, and good outpatient services, which not only treat patients, but also actively seek out others to treat early in their illnesses and which maintain registers of all patients.

Low overall admission rates in Eastern Europe reflect, then, widespread use of outpatient treatment programs in decentralized facilities. Although patterns of hospital utilization vary, the general trend, as a result of modern treatment methods, has been toward reducing the duration of hospital stay. According to Grof and Prokupek, the average period of hospitalization in Czechoslovakia was 262 days in 1955 and only 190 days in 1962. Associated with this trend has been an increase in readmission rates—a result of extending open-door programs as hospitals are increasingly used for acute problems. In Czechoslovakia the number of readmissions increased from 33.0 percent to 50.3 percent between 1958 and 1963. Shortened hospital stay, coupled with the increasing discharge rate, has had an overall effect of reducing crowding in hospitals.

PSYCHIATRIC TREATMENT

The enormous range of psychiatric treatments in the Communist countries partly reflects different theoretical orientations. Varying even from hospital to hospital, the approach to treatment in these countries is by and large a somatic one in which constitutional, genetic, and physical factors are all stressed. In parts of Eastern Europe, especially in Hungary and East Germany, the theories of Kretschmer, Kraepelin, Kleist, and Leonhard are most influential, whereas elsewhere the focus is on Pavlovian conditioning techniques. Physical treatment, including psychopharmaceutical agents, electroconvulsive shock therapy, and modified insulin, is widely emphasized.

The introduction of chlorpromazine and reserpine in the early 1950's, of numerous major and minor tranquilizing drugs, and, more recently, of antidepressants or psychic energizers has had as significant an effect in the Communist countries as in other parts of the world. Hospital practice has been immeasurably affected. These drugs have reduced the incidence of psychomotor agitation and aggressiveness, have made possible the elimination of mechanical restraints, and have facilitated the development of many of the open-door and community-oriented programs which characterize psychiatry today. Indeed, these drugs have become the major somatic therapy in the Communist countries. However, in many places—in Poland, for example—ECT is still the treatment of choice for involutional melancholia. In parts of the Soviet Union and in Bulgaria, where elimination of focal sepsis is stressed in getting patients into perfect physical condition, ECT and insulin coma treatment are still preferred. In Budapest regressive ECT and mechanical restraints are sometimes used instead of sedatives in excited cases. Lobotomy is everywhere illegal.

It is in conjunction with a number of other active measures that the new psychopharmaceutical agents are vigorously applied. Social rehabilitation through work therapy, for example, is very advanced in the Communist countries. A mentally-ill worker draws a disability pension for as long as he is unable to work and his family is cared for while he is ill. In the Soviet Union, workshops comprising complete industrial production units are available for inpatients as well as for outpatients. Patients receive full training and full industry-scale pay for their work. Notably, the emphasis on work therapy fits into the rationale of Communist society. In Marxist theory work is viewed as man's most important activity. It is felt that man's consciousness grows and his relations with other men develop within the framework of economic activities. According to the Soviet Constitution, work is a duty and a matter of honor.

Such methods of treatment as intensive, detailed, individual analysis, which cannot possibly become an instrument of wide social use, do not receive wide acceptance. Mild character difficulties are handled through social arrangement rather than through psychiatrists, and psychiatric facilities are devoted to those suffering most acutely.

In most places psychotherapy follows a medical model. Supporting and encouraging the patient, the doctor focuses on relieving symptoms rather than on effecting a basic personality change. Psychotherapists at the Bechterev Institute in Leningrad explicitly dissociate themselves from Freudian doctrine and combine a pedagogical approach with a view of the etiology of neuroses as bad education and bad habits. Thus they combine biological and psychological factors in a manner similar to that of Adolf Meyer. Treatment, called "rational therapy," consists of four phases. In the first, a protective phase involving pharmacological and electroshock-sleep treatment and hypnotic and other techniques, the idea is to establish an acceptable environmental situation. In the second phase, called "clarification," the patient is helped to see connections between his symptoms and his problems. The third phase is devoted to "reconstruction," or rebuilding, and new habits are consciously and actively sought. In the final, or training, phase the patient improves and perfects his newly acquired habits.

Psychotherapy is thus viewed as a process of reeducating the central nervous system by extinguishing pathologically conditioned connections and forming healthy new ones. Healthy mental processes are considered the result of a harmonious equilibrium between inhibition and excitation and between the first and second signal systems. A disruption of the latter impairs the capacity for abstract thought and is expressed clinically in disorganized behavior and thought. The therapeutic goal, then, is to inhibit pathological activity of the higher nervous centers and hence strengthen cortical control. To this end rest, relaxation, and suitably selected work are prescribed. In addition, persuasion, suggestion, autosuggestion, and hypnosis are believed to help mobilize the patient, his illness, and all the factors affecting it.

These general principles on which rational therapy is based seem to apply to other techniques of psychotherapy employed in Eastern Europe. In Bulgaria, for example, Krustnikov introduced a form of psychocatharsis called "reproduction psychotherapy," grounded in his theory concerning disturbed reflex activity of the psychons. This doctrine of the psychons, or units corresponding to the nervous system, was perhaps the most influential theory in Bulgarian psychiatry. Another technique, the "autogenic training" developed in East Germany, assumes the possibility of creating new conditioned reflexes. During the first stage of therapy intensive use is made of external suggestion, including hypnosis, to promote tranquilization and therapeutic sleep. In the second stage, occupational and musical therapy are used individually and in groups. In severe cases, especially in neurotic disturbances, autogenic training involves long-term psychotherapeutic sessions. Individual psychotherapy is used also to supplement the physiological treatment of psychoses and organic disorders.

In East Germany another form of therapy was initiated by Leonhard. This "individual therapy" relies heavily upon exercises to alter the patient's habits. In long sessions the therapist tries to convince his patient to execute each detail of the prescribed programs which vary with the patient's problems. In cases of hysterical neurosis, constant appeals are made to the patient's willpower. By contrast, a compulsive, tormented patient is assured that the therapist is acquainted with his profound sense of responsibility and his conscientiousness.

In the chapter on Czechoslovakia, Grof, Stuchlik, and Prokupek note that psychotherapy is there considered an indispensable technique which should, however, accompany other forms of therapy. Supportive psychotherapy, hypnosis, and autogenous training are all currently used. Although the Psychoanalytic Association, founded in Czechoslovakia before the war, was dissolved in 1950, dynamically oriented psychotherapy has become more prominent in the last decade. At the new center of dynamic psychotherapy set up at Charles University in Prague, neurotic patients participate in various forms of psychotherapy. In Yugoslavia, dynamically oriented psychotherapy presently flourishes. In Zagreb, Stepan Betlheim, a pupil of Paul Schilder, directs the only center for psychotherapy in Eastern Europe which follows the classical psychoanalytic approach. In Poland, where it is increasingly used, nonphysicians have been trained as therapists. In a recently established neurotic treatment center, group psychotherapy is practiced and, as Gnat points out, training analyses are required in order for the psychotherapist to "get an insight into his individual problems, control his attitudes toward patients and limit his own emotional attitudes in the interpretation of the characteristic features of patients' personalities." This view, so atypical in Eastern Europe, underscores the extent to which diversity exists even in generally uniform systems.

While neuroses are considered psychogenic and are generally treated with some form of rational therapy, other methods are applied as well: massage, remedial exercises, drugs, supportive therapy, mud therapy and other forms of balneology, physiotherapy, and inhalation therapy. A change of environment is also commonly advocated. If so, the patient is usually sent away from his family to a sanitorium for a twenty-one-day rest period.

Associated with rational psychotherapy is a public health view that neurotic reactions are more frequent under conditions of social decay and stagnation. Prevention of neuroses is thus related to the solution of housing problems, the emancipation of women, proper education of the youth, help for preschool and school groups alike, special work campaigns, and the growth of various sports among the youth. Mental hygiene focuses on vocational placement, rehabilitation of disabled veterans, control of psychiatric disorders through early diagnosis, the fight against alcoholism, guidance in sexual matters, and other programs of this nature.

The integration of public health and medical approaches is perhaps best exemplified in the treatment of alcoholism. In Poland, for instance, special provisions for alcoholics were introduced in April, 1956. The measures included compulsory treatment of alcoholics, legal protection and care of their families, and the establishment of "sober-down homes." In 1959, provision was made for setting up district therapeutic institutions and municipal outpatient departments for alcoholics. In some form, measures both to control alcoholics and to care for their families have been instituted in the other Communist countries as well.

Psychiatric treatment in China, according to Bermann's account, has much in common with treatment in Eastern Europe. The treatment of psychasthenia, for example, combines Pavlov's mixture of caffeine and bromide with small doses of insulin, Chinese herbs, hormones, nerve tonics, novocaine, electric sleep, physical and respiratory exercises, and iron therapy. In addition, patients are treated with a combination of directive, didactic, individual, and group psychotherapy directed especially at the development of a moral and social conscience.

ORGANIZATION OF RESEARCH AND PERSONNEL

Extensive psychiatric research tends to reflect a developed state of psychiatry, although it is clear that research can thrive even in a country which has not met all the problems of service. Where research is done, it indicates not only the theoretical orientation of the psychiatrists but also the availability of statistical reporting systems, research money, and of personnel. It should be emphasized that in Eastern Europe, psychiatry and neurology have been combined in the university curricula, in the programs of many hospitals, and in the training of specialists. Logically, this combination has stimulated interest in mental disorders of organic origin, and research in neuroanatomy, neuropathology, neurophysiology, biochemistry, and genetics tends to predominate.

In Eastern European countries scientific and technological research is centrally directed by governmental committees which assign priorities and select areas in which progress is most important and in which men and materials should be concentrated. The Academies of Sciences plan the specific research and direct its execution. Hence, research programs in particular institutes or centers tend to be components of long-term plans which are coordinated with the government's economic plans. Thus, the Soviet Union has five-year plans in psychiatry as well as in other areas of endeavor, such as economics. For example, in 1955, psychiatrists were urged to study schizophrenia, neuroinfections, cerebral vascular diseases, and the administrative problems of research.

In 1959 the Academy of Sciences made some effort to decentralize the system of administering and planning Soviet scientific research. This reform was intended to give individual scientific institutions greater influence in deciding what research work was to be carried on. Under the new plan a small number of the most important scientific problems would continue to be approved at the central government level, and would be embodied in a document to be called "Basic Directions of Scientific Research in the U.S.S.R." Once approved, each basic problem would be handled by a scientific council of leading scientists and heads of research institutes, with the decisions on special research projects being made by research institutions or by government agencies financing particular research areas.

This pattern of decentralization is being followed in other Eastern European countries. In Bulgaria, the Academy of Sciences focuses on the experimental encephalitides; the psychopharmacology group of the Sofia Faculty of Medicine concentrates on exogenous-toxic psychoses; and other institutes concern themselves with schizophrenia, forensic psychiatry, neuroses, psychopathies, and psychotherapy.

Much of the research activity has developed in recent years, as exemplified by the work of the Psychiatric Institute (Bohmice) in Prague, which started functioning in January, 1961, as a research institute of the Ministry of Health and as a center for all of Czechoslovakia's psychiatric research. Informed by wide contacts with both Eastern and Western countries, the Institute's extensive range of research has become perhaps the most striking feature of contemporary psychiatry in Czechoslovakia. Indeed, studies actively pursued are so diverse as to include measurement of catecholamines and their metabolites in the urine, the distribution of mental disorders in urban areas, and the investigation of new psychotropic drugs. Histochemical, sensory-deprivation, and physiological studies are among the other investigations being carried on, further illustrating that methodological sophistication of the highest calibre is in keeping with Czechoslovakia's outstanding tradition of scientific psychiatry.

In Poland, where research has been dominated by the physiological approach already popular before World War II, investigations currently utilize such methods as electroencephalography, galvanic skin responses, and electrophoresis. Research ranges from conditioning by unconscious stimulation to drug toxicity in animals and even to social-psychiatric investigations of the effect of migration to new towns. In fact, Polish research now includes studies whose orientation is psychological, descriptive, and phenomenological, as well as physiological.

The unique feature of contemporary Rumanian psychiatry is its research on the endocrine aspects of psychiatric disorders. Initiated at the end of the nineteenth century by Professor Constantine I. Parhon, work in this area has been intensive. At present, the basic biological substratum of both the severe and less severe disorders is being actively investigated with biochemical, immunological, electroencephalogic, and other techniques. Csiky hypothesizes that schizophrenia is a process which affects certain morpho-functional structures, weakened by predisposing, favoring and provoking factors. Prinzei, on the other hand, regards schizophrenia as due to an encephalodistrophy of an endo-exogenous nature.

In China, where the major psychiatric problem is schizophrenia, research has been largely organically oriented. Most notable have been studies of acetaldelyde, the metabolism of amino acids, and electroencephalography.

Epidemiological research is especially advanced in the Soviet Union, Poland, Czechoslovakia, and Bulgaria. These countries' extensive networks of clinics make large-scale epidemiological studies particularly feasible. However, studies of this nature are also conducted in Yugoslavia, where services are just beginning to be developed on an extensive basis. In fact, the most interesting feature of Yugoslavian psychiatry today is the great sensitivity to the changing pattern of mental illness illustrated in these studies. A relationship has been found between industrialization and urbanization and an increase of mental disorders, suicide rates, absenteeism, alcoholism and delinquency. Although these increased rates are partly due to better detection and improved diagnostic approaches, they undoubtedly reflect the impact of social change on the mental health of the society.

At present the Institute of Psychiatry in Moscow is engaged in a follow-up study to ascertain the natural course of all forms of schizophrenia in and out of the hospital. It is currently thought that cases never treated in the hospital are of the same three basic forms (distinguished by Sneznevsky) as those seen in hospital cases, but that clinical courses differ.

Epidemiological studies are also used, at least in the Soviet Union, to advise the Ministry of Health about district bed requirements, which depend upon the distribution of age groups and types of illness in the population. Again, it is through the extensive network of clinics that people, once registered, can be followed for many years.

The impact of bureaucracy is also evident in the career lines of physicians. The individual's profession is determined (partly at the secondary-school level) not only by his abilities and interests, but also by the needs of the state. From then on, his education and training are coordinated by a central body responsible for meeting the needs of the society. All members of the medical profession are expected to enter government service. Every doctor is assigned either to a district with a specified number of patients or to a hospital. These assignments are made after consideration of geographical location and areas of specialization. A doctor selects his specialty on the basis of the required quota. There is evidence that these patterns are changing and that individual choice plays a greater role in all phases of an individual's career.

DISCUSSION

Prevention and public health probably form the dominant themes of psychiatry in the Communist countries. Undoubtedly, this orientation is tied up with the belief that psychiatric illness is amenable to prophylactic measures and large-scale efforts not unlike those used to control infectious and contagious diseases. Indeed, the prevention of many diseases by altering environmental pathogenetic factors provides a model compatible with the Marxist focus on social environmental factors in the individual's development.

It should be emphasized that many preventable psychiatric disorders are in fact secondary to infectious, parasitic, and toxic agents. In Eastern Europe, psychiatrists are very closely allied to the medical specialties and encounter some of these disorders often enough to support a general preventive orientation. Since a number of these conditions are associated with poverty, poor nutrition, inadequate housing, and poor sanitation, it is only natural for psychiatrists to think in terms of preventing them by environmental manipulation. It is only a step further to think in terms of preventing psychogenic disorders by the same kinds of environmental manipulation. Indeed, it is very difficult for the psychiatrist so oriented to view disorders as deriving from intrapsychic factors.

Many people are interested in the impact of automation, migration, and other social events that seem to be connected with a greater incidence of psychiatric disturbance. Again, one should point to Eastern Europe's rehabilitative and preventive programs in hospitals, in industrial plants, in factories, and on farms, which have long been key aspects of these countries' programs of psychiatry. Thus occupational, family, and social roles are stressed in the treatment of patients, and great efforts are made to keep people functioning as long as possible in the community, and to reserve mental-hospital beds largely for neurotics who may benefit from environmental change.

In addition to a public health approach to psychiatry, Eastern

European countries emphasize continuity of care and comprehensive treatment programs. Epidemiological registers are assiduously maintained so that health services and the problems of community diagnosis can be continually evaluated. Thus it is possible to assess the magnitude of a problem in different communities and to plan programs on this basis. Numbers, types, and classification of admissions by age, sex, and nationality, and diagnostic frequency distributions are obtainable through the central registries. These data enable psychiatrists to assess the needs of the population and the different kinds of programs that must be set up. Since not all cases go to the hospital, it is possible to compare the treated with the untreated population and also to determine how these two groups are differentially distributed in the general population. With the central registries it is also possible to investigate the dispositions of individuals with different diagnoses and to follow them through their progress into different facilities and aftercare programs. In addition, one can determine individual risks and sometimes even the etiology of the various disorders.

Within a public health orientation, emphasis is greatest on using those treatments which have proven most effective and which can be most readily applied to large portions of the population. Although psychotherapy is not particularly adapted to this orientation, drug therapy, sleep therapy, and shock therapy are appropriate. Individual symptomatic treatment is certainly valued, but maximum utilization of facilities and personnel is the order of the day. People working in the mental health field can be continually relocated so that a maximum number are operating in the area where the maximum need exists.

Some of the most progressive developments in the hospital treatment of psychiatric patients have occurred since World War II. More and more efforts are being made to reduce the necessity of certification, to increase the resources of community services and general hospitals, and to discourage custodial patterns in mental hospitals.

A striking feature of many mental hospitals in the Communist countries is the increased use of part-time hospital programs along with community facilities. Treatment programs are arranged so that patients can be maintained at home on a domiciliary-visit basis or be treated by physical or occupational therapy at the day hospital. Naturally enough, these programs lead to reduced hospital admission rates.

Patients are provided with continuity of care in and out of the hospital. Because of an active system of home visits by doctors and social workers, patients not only are seen in the early stages of illness when preventive measures can still be employed, but also receive continuous care by the same individuals before, during, and after admission. Time in the hospital can be shortened with less risk than previously.

Day units permit earlier discharge from the hospital and a setting for thorough aftercare. Treatment facilities are concentrated in the community and patients are admitted to the hospital, on a short-term basis, only when community or home resources prove inadequate for therapy and management. Among the facilities which operate solely on a daily basis are day hospitals, geriatric day centers, outpatient departments of hospitals, some psychiatric hospitals, and industrial-rehabilitation units. Patients with physical, mental, or social handicaps undergo rehabilitation courses in clerical work, carpentry, tool-making, or the use of industrial machinery. Trained workers supervise the work, provide vocational guidance, and assist in job placement. In accord with their focus on public health, the Communist countries have developed a great number of important treatment and rehabilitative measures that can be utilized on a large scale.

The chapters that follow cover a wide range of subjects, each of which could be separately studied and analyzed. At the same time, various analyses of the volume as a whole could be suggested to different readers depending on their interests and disciplines. In this introductory chapter, I have attempted to outline only the major issues and implications of the material.

A Note About the Sources

A variety of material was read in the course of preparing this volume to provide background information against which to study the submitted chapters. The bulk of available reading material focused primarily on the Soviet Union. Some of the published political analyses contained information which has been referred to in the introductory chapter. The most important of these sources are included in the following bibliography. Of greater interest, however, are the references cited in the respective chapters; the bulk of those references are unfamiliar to Western psychiatrists.

Bibliography

J. ARONSON AND M. G. FIELD: Mental Health Programming in the Soviet Union, *Amer. J. Orthopsychiat.*, 34:913–924 (1964).

YE. D. ASHURKOV, A. B. SHEVELEV, AND S. M. DANYUSHEVSKIY: Coordination of Scientific Research on Public Health in the Socialist Countries, *Sovetskoye Zdavookhraneniye* (Soviet Public Health), 19 (8):6–13 (1960).

T. A. BAN AND J. ST. LAURENT: Quelques aspects theoriques de la psychiatrie en Russie et autres fays de l'Europe de l'Est, *Canadian Psychiatric Association Journal*, 6 (2):88–95.

M. I. BARSUKOV: Problems in the Study of the Theory and History of Medicine in the USSR in the Light of Decisions of the 21st Congress of the Communist Party of the Soviet Union, *Sovetskaya Meditsina* (Soviet Medicine), 23 (7):3–12 (1959).

R. A. BAUER, A. INKELES, AND C. KLUCKHOHN: "How the Soviet System Works," Vintage Books, New York, 1956.

Z. K. BRZEZINSKI: "Soviet Bloc—Unity and Conflict," Praeger, New York, 1963.

V. BUSEK: "Czechoslovakia," Praeger, New York, 1957.

R. F. BYRNES: "Yugoslavia," Praeger, New York, 1957.

CHAO I-PING: Communist China's Achievements in Pavlov's Theory During the Past Decade, *Sheng-wu-hsueh T'ung-pao* (Biology Bulletin), (10) 468–471 (October, 1959).

K. DABROWSKI, T. GNAT, A. JAROSZEWSKI, AND A. JUS: "Assistance psychiatrique en Pologne," Comite Polonais de L'Annee Mondiale de la Sante Mentale, Etabli d'apres les documents de la Conference Nationale des Psychiatres Polonais a Branice en juin 1960.

L. A. D. DELLIN: "Bulgaria," Praeger, New York, 1957.

M. G. FIELD: "Doctor and Patient in Soviet Russia," Harvard University Press, Cambridge, Mass., 1957.

——: Soviet Community Mental Health Services and Work Therapy: A Report of Two Visits, *Community Mental Health Journal*, 1 (1):81–90, 1965.

—— AND J. ARONSON: The Institutional Framework of Soviet Psychiatry, *J. Nerv. Ment. Dis.*, 138:305–322, 1964.

STEPHEN FISHER-GALATI: "Rumania," Praeger, New York, 1957.

Forty Years of Soviet Medicine, *Le Concours Medical* (The Medical Forum) [Paris], 189–196 (January, 1960).

O. HALECKI: "Poland," Praeger, New York, 1957.

Health Services in the USSR, Public Health Papers, (3), WHO, Geneva, 1960.

E. HELMREICH: "Hungary," Praeger, New York, 1957.

I. L. HOROWITZ: "Three Worlds of Development—the Theory and Practice of International Stratification," Oxford University Press, New York, 1966.

A. A. HUTSCHNECKER: Medicine and Psychiatry in the Union of Soviet

Socialist Republics, *Transactions N.Y. Academy of Science,* 22:585 (1960).

N. V. IVANOV: The Problem of the Theory of Soviet Group Psychotherapy. Psychiatry in the USSR and Czechoslovakia, *Zhurnal Nevropatologii i Psikhiatrii* (Journal of Neuropathology and Psychiatry), 60 (10) 1342–1351; 1391–1396 (1960).

Z. JAROSZEWSKI: *Bulletyn Statystyczny* (Statistical Bulletin) *Psychiatry, 1956–1959,* Ministry of Health and Social Welfare, Warsaw, 1963.

L. B. KALINOWSKY: Impressions of Soviet Psychiatry, *Comprehensive Psychiatry,* 1:35–41 (1960).

A. H. KAPLAN: Trends in Soviet Psychiatry, *Mental Hygiene,* 46:20–30 (1962).

I. A. KHRISTOFOROVA: Experience in Studying the Incidence of Disease Among the Population of Certain Areas, *Tadzhikistan Health* (Stalinabad), (7) (3):11–15 (May/June, 1960).

N. S. KLINE: The Organization of Psychiatric Care and Psychiatric Research in the USSR, *Ann. N.Y. Acad. Sci.,* 84:147–224 (1960).

————, M. G. FIELD, AND J. ARONSON: Soviet Psychiatric Nomenclature, *Amer. J. Psychiat.,* 118:178–180 (1961).

P. KOPORIC AND N. PERSIC: Polyclinical and Outpatient Psychiatric Services in Croatia, *Lijecnicki Bjesnik,* 83 (5):445–458 (1961).

C. KOUPERNIK: A propos de trois ouvrages neuro-psychiatriques Russes, *Evolution Psychiatrique,* 25:635–648 (1960).

S. V. KURASHOV: Improvement of Medical Service and the Preservation of Health in the USSR, *Meditsinskiy Rabotnik* (Medical Worker), 23 (98):1–3 (1960).

D. LAZURE: The Family and Youth in New China: Psychiatric Observations, *The Canadian Medical Assoc. Jour.,* 86:179–183 (January 27, 1962).

Z. M. LEBENSOHN: Impressions of Soviet Psychiatry, *A.M.A. Archives of Neuro. and Psychiat.,* 80:735–751 (1958).

J. L. MORENO: Psychiatric Encounter in Soviet Russia, *Progress in Psychotherapy,* 5:1–24 (1960).

V. M. MOROZOV: Depth Psychology and Psychiatry, *Zhurnal Nervopatologii i Psikhiatrii* (Journal of Neuropathology and Psychiatry), 58 (11): 1399–1406 (1958).

A. F. K. ORGANSKI: "The Stages of Political Development," Alfred A. Knopf, New York, 1965.

D. E. PENTONY (ed.): "Soviet Behavior in World Affairs," Chandler Publishing Company, San Francisco, 1962.

O. V. PEROV: Criticism of Freudian Teachings with Respect to the Assessment of Occupational Activities, *Sovetskoye Adavookhraneniye* (Soviet Public Health), (11):15–20 (1960).

S. A. PETRUSHEVSKIY AND N. S. MANSUROV: The American Way of Life Before the Court of Materialist Psychology and Psychiatry, *Voprosy Filosofil* (Problems of Philosophy), (4):156–161 (1959).

A. M. RAPOPORT: On the Composition and Disposition of Patients in USSR

Psychiatric Institutions, *Zhur. Nevropatolog. i Pskihiatrii imeni S.S. Korsakova* (Korsakov Journal of Neuropathology and Psychiatry), 57 (1):95–103 (1957).

G. RAZRAN: Soviet Psychology and Psychophysiology, *Science*, 128:1187–1195 (1958).

Research Institutes of Chinese Traditional Medicine: Achievements in Perpetuating and Promoting Chinese Traditional Medicine, *Ch'ing-chu Chien-kuo Shih-chou-nien I-hseuh Ch-eng chiu Lun-wen Chi*, 1:291–298 (December, 1959).

K. ROWINSKI: Scientists and Research Work in the Medical Academies of Poland, *Polski Tygodnik Lekarski* (Polish Medical Weekly), 15: 1321–1327; 1366–1369 (1960).

H. SETON-WATSON: "The East European Revolution," Praeger, New York, 1962.

S. SKENDI (ed.): "Albania," Praeger, New York, 1958.

Y. Y. SVIRINOVSKIY AND B. V. SHOSTAKOVICH: Compulsory Treatment As One Method of Preventing the Repeated Socially Dangerous Actions of Mentally Deranged Patients, *Sudebno-Meditsinskaya Espertiza* (Forensic Medical Expertise), (3):47–49 (1959).

R. B. WINN: "Psychotherapy in the Soviet Union," Grove Press, New York, 1962.

J. WORTIS: "Soviet Psychiatry," Williams & Wilkins, Baltimore, 1950.

———: The Thaw in Soviet Psychiatry, *Amer. J. Psychiat.*, 119:586–588 (1962).

CHAPTER TWO

Soviet Psychiatry

BY
DR. A. G. GALACH'YAN

AS IN OTHER COUNTRIES, the history of the development of psychiatric theories in Russia is closely related to that of national culture and law. Although for the most part paralleling the development of this discipline in other European nations, Russian psychiatry has had a number of distinctive features which have left a special mark on it, as manifested in the attitude of large segments of the populace toward the mentally ill, in the manner in which such persons are cared for, and in the entire character of the system of psychiatric aid in the Soviet Union from its reorganization on scientific principles down to the present day. During the early phases of Russian history, when the oppressed masses were cruelly exploited by the ruling aristocracy, the involuntary sympathy and concern of the people were extended to the many even more helpless and humble feeble-minded and so-called "transcendents," the majority of whom were chronic mental illness cases; their disjointed, irrational ravings often reflected the hopelessly difficult position of the impoverished populace and the greed and cruelty of their oppressors. The incomprehensible oddity of the statements of the mentally ill, foreign to the everyday experience and

notions of the populace, was, as in the Western nations, accepted on the
religious-mystic level. However, in contrast to Westerners, who usually
attached a demonological significance to all this, the Russian populace
regarded it as an unusual, extremely severe form of religious transport
manifested in a type of insanity, an extremely severe form of prolonged
epithymia. Despite the fact that, as a result of the general breakdown
of law during the Middle Ages, the army of fools, pilgrims, wanderers,
and cripples had been swelled by clearly parasitic, adventuristic elements
who gambled on the charity and compassion of the population toward the
sick, the general attitude toward the mentally ill remained constant, and
a concerned humane approach became traditional in Russia.

A frequent concomitant of the delusory experiences of the mentally
ill is the idea of possession by an "evil force," which produces an "evil
spirit," etc., in the affected individual; this furnishes a basis for regarding
sufferers from delusions as possessed, bedeviled, or deranged, or as magi-
cians or clairvoyants who have "sold their souls to the devil." The populace considered members of the former group as sufferers without pain,
in final analysis as sick persons who had to be liberated from evil by
prayer and fasting. While the Inquisition raged in the West and tens of
thousands of mentally ill persons and hysterics died at the stake when its
tribunals found the "devil's stigmata" on their bodies, the history of
Russian psychiatry knew none of these horrors. Isolated cases in which
the mentally ill were burnt at the stake did occur in Russia, but such
cruelties toward mentally deficient individuals usually took place when
behavioral improprieties or irrational statements touched on religious
dogma or were directed at the ecclesiastical or governmental aristocracy;
cruel punishments of this type were generally inflicted on persons suspected of practicing black magic. Punishments had the character of
administrative measures for coping with dissatisfied persons and individuals
dangerous to the existing governmental order or to those about them.

In the distant past, monasteries were the first refuges for the mentally
ill in Russia, especially for "violent" patients, i.e., disturbed, aggressive
individuals. As a rule, only such persons were, in keeping with the laws
of the times, subjected to violent, crude restraints, sometimes for protracted
periods. As the patient's agitated state abated, the emphasis in handling
him shifted to soothing conversations with the monks, exhortation, prayer,
religious rituals, etc. The residents of monasteries were repeatedly re-
minded of the need for a humane attitude toward and spiritual guidance
of the mentally ill. From the latter half of the eighteenth century onward,

monasteries lost their importance in the care of these individuals, although some continued to be places of imprisonment for persons especially dangerous to the ecclesiastical and civil authorities until the late nineteenth century.

In some cases Russian monasteries, just as those in other nations, exploited the fact that they sheltered the mentally ill to attract pilgrims and financial contributions: The ecclesiastical authorities of the monastery would capitalize on the grotesque, disjointed, sometimes senseless statements and peculiar behavior of the patients by advertising them as persons with the aforementioned special gifts of clairvoyance and prophecy.

The first special institution for mental patients in Russia, the "Special Home," was built in Novgorod in 1762; a second institution, the "Home for the Insane," was built in Petersburg seventeen years later. In 1775, as a result of a governmental edict establishing Boards of Public Welfare with their own funds in each province, the responsibility of caring for the mentally ill and feeble-minded was transferred to these organizations. In addition to therapeutic institutions and pharmacies, the Boards took charge of all orphanages, workhouses, and poorhouses. Institutions similar to the Petersburg Home for the Insane were subsequently built in other provincial cities, and departments for the mentally ill were opened in provincial hospitals.

At about the time when the county public medical services were organized (1864) the Boards of Public Welfare included fifty-four "homes for the insane" among their charges. The transfer of the existing therapeutic institutions and funds from the Boards to the autonomous control of the county and municipal administrations marked the beginning of the reorganization of older psychiatric institutions and the establishment of new ones based on scientific principles. The intensive construction of large county psychiatric hospitals, which coincided with the brief improvement in social conditions during the 1860's, was unfortunately impeded at every turn by the paucity of funds received by the county administrations from the Boards of Public Welfare and also by the general lack of material resources in the county and municipal social organizations. Nevertheless, by the end of the 1880's the number of psychiatric institutions in Russia was double the aforementioned number of "homes for the insane."*

---

* Numerous data pertaining to the era of Kievan Russia and the Moscow government are presented in the exhaustive monograph *An Outline of the History of Russian Psychiatry* by the noted Soviet psychiatrist T. I. Yudin (1951), to which we refer the reader.

During the last quarter of the nineteenth century the free county medical and psychiatric services, which reached the residents of the most remote corners of Russia, attracted all the progressively minded young physicians of the nation. This phenomenon further extended and expanded the concerned, humane attitude toward the mentally ill in Russia. Through their booths at the Dresden World's Fair of 1897 the county medical services attracted the attention of physicians from other countries. In the oft-repeated opinion of the noted hygienist F. F. Erisma, this achievement of the Russian public medical service was unique, having no counterpart in any other nation. Even the political reaction in Russia during the 1880's and following the revolution in 1905 could not destroy the progressive traditions of the county psychiatric services, and their most advanced ideas survived to see the Great October Revolution.

The Russian public psychiatric service was not only able, within the comparatively short space of twenty to twenty-five years, to reorganize the "homes for the insane" and the departments for psychiatric patients at provincial general hospitals, to build a network of large new regional psychiatric hospitals, and to carry on a continuous, tenacious struggle to protect the personal rights of the mentally ill, it was also able to eliminate the "hot shirt," strait jacket, and similar cruel restraints from Russian psychiatric institutions. Connolly's nonrestraint system, which S. S. Korsakov introduced at a small private psychiatric clinic in Moscow during the early 1880's, was quickly adopted by other Russian psychiatrists as something self-evident and soon became customary procedure in most psychiatric hospitals. By the end of the century there was perhaps not a single psychiatric institution in Russia which still employed the crude restraints mentioned above. Such was not the case for all psychiatric hospitals in the West at the time. This indubitable achievement of Russian psychiatrists can be attributed both to the extraordinary moral and scientific authority of S. S. Korsakov and, perhaps, primarily, to the traditionally concerned, humane attitude of the populace toward the mentally ill.

The vast areas with predominantly rural populations served by the provincial hospitals made it necessary to bring psychiatric services nearer to the people through decentralization and to establish a close relationship between the psychiatric hospitals and the regions' general medical services. Since patients discharged from the psychiatric hospitals actually were under the subsequent care of rural physicians, continuous, on-the-spot medical observation and treatment could be ensured only when the doctor was interested in the patient's fate. Farming was the principal occupation

of the overwhelming majority of the populace, and from the very outset
the regional psychiatric services placed great emphasis on treating patients
through organized agricultural labor. This, to a considerable extent, explains their tendency to build new psychiatric hospitals not in or near
cities but at some distance from them, in heavily agrarian areas where it
was possible to organize agricultural work for the patients on a large scale.
It is consequently not accidental that it was in Novgorod County that this
type of psychiatric institution was first set up on a major scale in Russia.
The psychiatric colony in Novgorod County was established by Doctor
E. F. Andriol and involved a broad range of agricultural work as occupational therapy; it was patterned on the German psychiatric colony founded
eighteen years earlier at Alt-Scherbitz.

Many of the ideas and innovations of Russian social psychiatrists
naturally could not be realized under the conditions of Czarist Russia;
realization became possible only after the October Socialist Revolution.

Throughout all the phases of its scientific development Russian psychiatry was based on materialistic concepts of the nature of mental illnesses. Psychiatric hospitals were headed by physicians from the very
beginning of the period of intensive construction, since even the broad
masses of the populace recognized the mentally ill as sick persons requiring
medical treatment, despite the religious-mystical interpretations placed on
the manifestations and origins of psychosis. Physicians learned materialistic
concepts while still at medical school from their instructors in the theory
of mental illness. These instructors were not at that time specialists but
were drawn from among the professors of other departments of the faculty.
For all their unfamiliarity with the discipline in question, these casual
instructors in psychiatry based their explanations on the scientific judg-
ments they were accustomed to utilize. It may be that such an attitude
toward psychiatry, albeit a detached one, on the part of certain of the most
talented Moscow professors and clinicians of the first half of the nineteenth century helped lead them to the notion of a close relationship between the psychic and the somatic, the problem of neurism, which was
later so brilliantly developed by I. M. Sechenov and especially by I. P.
Pavlov. Perhaps this was the reason why the "psychiatric dualism" which
long held sway in Western psychiatry, particularly in that of Germany,
with its protracted struggle between psychic and somatic psychiatrists, was
always foreign to Russian psychiatry.

The next characteristic feature of Russian and Soviet psychiatry is the
extremely close relationship between theory and practice. The initial de-

velopment of scientific psychiatry and, for some time, its subsequent progress were achieved by practical clinical psychiatrists through their observations of the mentally ill in therapeutic institutions. Ts. Kh. Kandinskiy, a physician at the Petersburg Hospital, conducted the classical investigation of pseudohallucination, which subsequently came to be known as the Kandinskiy-Clerambault syndrome. It is advantageous to distinguish the works of practical psychiatrists from treatises and textbooks on psychiatry by university professors who, in addition to their basic specialties, were involved in teaching the theory of mental illness to medical students. The works of the latter had an exceptionally compilative character and naturally were considerably inferior to those of the former, which cited the results of years of personal clinical observation and experience. A tendency toward experimental clinical investigations became traditional in Russian psychiatry, and two major psychiatric schools developed, one in Petersburg (Leningrad) and one in Moscow, during the last quarter of the nineteenth century.

The clinical trend was especially clear in S. S. Korsakov's psychiatric school in Moscow (The Korsakov School), Korsakov having been a student of A. Ya. Kozhevnikov, the founder of neuropathology. In 1887, shortly after the university psychiatric clinic had been built in Moscow, the department of psychiatry was separated from the department of nervous diseases. The Leningrad psychiatric school was headed by the "father of Russian psychiatry," I. M. Balinskiy, a "pure psychiatrist." There was a single department of nervous and mental illnesses in Leningrad until 1916; a separate department of psychiatry was established after V. M. Bekhterev retired. It seems to us that the prolonged period for which the two disciplines were combined in a single department is attributable to a certain neurological bias on the part of the members of the Leningrad school, a tendency which has persisted down to the present. These two psychiatric schools produced a substantial number of leading Russian psychiatrists, the majority of whom founded their own independent schools.

To the younger generation of Russian psychiatrists fell the task of developing a Soviet psychiatry after the October Socialist Revolution. Soviet psychiatrists set about answering the urgent demands of Russian psychiatry, which it was impossible to satisfy under the conditions of the Czarist regime but which now called for realization in the light of the new social attitudes in the nation. The prophylactic trend in Soviet psychiatry, as in all Soviet medicine, necessitated the prompt organization of a network of outpatient centers to bring psychiatric care to the populace. A regional psychiatric service was set up in Moscow in 1919 and similar services were later established in other large cities. The functions of these services included complete care of psychiatric patients who remained with their families, creation of the most favorable possible domestic and other living conditions for such patients, protection of their personal interests and rights, and, when necessary, provision of a fixed monthly allotment to their families. While carrying out medical observation of the mentally ill of the district and providing them with therapeutic aid, the regional psychiatrists sent all patients whose mental condition deteriorated to psychiatric hospitals for institutional care. With the organization in the same year of the Moscow regional network of neuropsychiatric sanitariums for patients with borderline conditions, the regional psychiatrists became responsible for those of the sanitarium patients who had been recommended for further observation and treatment upon their discharge. As the number of neurological sanitariums increased, their medical staffs were augmented by psychiatrist-physicians, so that the concepts of clinical psychiatry came to be applied to an ever greater extent to borderline cases. The increased workload of the regional psychiatrists and the need for dynamic observation of patients and establishment of dispensary services eventually resulted in the reorganization of the existing system into a network of neurological-psychiatric clinics with even broader prophylactic responsibilities.

Soviet psychiatrists devoted a great deal of effort to decentralizing psychiatric facilities and reorganizing the network of "major psychiatric" institutions. Since the large regional psychiatric hospitals which supposedly served vast areas were capable of caring only for the residents of the portion of the region nearest each hosptal, it became necessary to open several smaller hospitals in the more remote areas. The building of psychiatric institutions in isolated regions of the national republics, which were largely neglected in this respect under the Czarist regime, became an especially pressing problem; an enormous amount of work was done in the construction of new institutions and in the reconstruction of the few pre-Revolutionary ones in these areas. In the early 1930's many psychiatric hospitals throughout the Soviet Union were converted to true therapeutic institutions by freeing the beds previously occupied by chronic patients, who required hospitalization in a different type of institution. Patients with acute psychotic conditions could be promptly and actively treated only with the facilities available at large, well-equipped psychiatric hospitals. To care for persons convalescing after an intensive course of therapy and for patients whose mental condition did not require confinement in restrictive therapeutic institutions, sanitarium branches were opened at psychiatric hospitals and neuropsychiatric clinics were established at neuropsychiatric hospitals and dispensaries. Psychiatric departments were organized at some large regional medical hospitals to handle cases of acute psychosis arising during the course of various infectious somatic diseases, after surgery, etc. The scope of this article does not permit us to consider this topic in greater detail, but we should point out one further achievement of Soviet psychiatry.

To bring psychiatric aid closer to the populace, Soviet psychiatrists (M. A. Dzhagarov, et al.) established a new form of semi-hospital, semi-clinical service, the *day ward*, which is set up as a special division of a psychiatric hospital. The patient spends the entire day, from early morning until evening, in this ward under a therapeutic regimen, receiving the necessary treatment, particularly psychotherapeutic aid, engaging in occupational therapy and cultural amusements, and being kept on a strict, full-valued diet; only in the evening is he permitted to return home to his family for the night.

In order to permit more thorough study of the problems associated with the operation of the network of prophylactic dispensaries, other outpatient facilties, and minor psychiatric clinics, the State Scientific Research Institute of Neuropsychiatric Prophylaxis was organized in 1925 on the basis of the State Neuropsychiatric Dispensary, which had already been in existence in Moscow for several years. L. M. Rozenshteyn, an enthusiastic advocate of the prophylactic-dispensary trend in psychiatry, was chosen to head the Institute, and Yu. V. Kannabikh, the scientific adviser and consultant to the large Moscow regional network of neuropsychiatric sanitariums, participated actively in its work.

The considerable scientific achievements of the Institute of Neuropsychiatric Prophylaxis in the clinical recognition and prophylaxis of latent forms of psychosis and borderline conditions were undoubtedly somewhat devalued by the methodological errors committed both in clinical psychopathological investigations and in psychoprophylactic and psychohygienic work. Sufficient attention was not always paid to the special features of the studies conducted by the Institute's dispensaries; no distinction was made among different groups of working data, which led to an incorrect application of psychopathological and diagnostic concepts taken from the field of "major" psychiatry to symptoms only remotely reminiscent of true psychiatric phenomena and mechanisms. All this naturally could not but have an unfavorable influence on psychohygienic and psychoprophylactic practice. As was the case at one time in child psychiatry, a deviation from strict clinical views and from a disciplined clinical way of thinking led to the unjustified application of biological concepts and criteria to phenomena caused by factors of an essentially social nature.

Psychiatric-research institutes were opened also in other cities. Some of them served all of Russia, whereas others served only individual republics or regions; the former accordingly occupied themselves with solving the central problems of theoretical and clinical psychiatry, the latter were more concerned with theoretical, clinical, organizational, and practical problems at the local level. Psychoneurological institutes were established in Leningrad (The V. M. Bekhterev Institute), as well as at Khar'kov, Kiev, Odessa, Baku, Tbilisi, Dnepropetrovsk, Tula, and other centers. Certain of these institutes were later closed as ineffective in line with the expansion of those in nearby cities. In 1920, even before the founding of the Institute of Neuropsychiatric Prophylaxis, the V. P. Serbskiu Institute of Forensic Psychiatry was established in Moscow; the P. B. Gannushkin Municipal Psychiatric Research Institute was founded in 1933; and the Institute of Psychiatry of the Academy of Medical Sciences U.S.S.R. in 1944. Psychiatric departments were also organized at the Institutes for Evaluation of Working Capacity and Working Conditions of the Commissariats of Social Security in Moscow, Leningrad, and the Ukraine.

THEORY

The expansion of Soviet psychiatry from the psychiatric hospitals into the broad field of borderline conditions, and the bringing of psychiatric help to new groups of patients, raised new theoretical and practical problems. Specifically required were the development of a clinical methodology for use in sanitariums, psychotherapeutic, psychohygienic, and psychoprophylactic techniques, and occupational therapy methods for institutions for borderline cases. The creation of a new, independent branch of clinical psychiatry, that dealing with children and adolescents, also posed a number of new problems for Soviet psychiatry; pre-Revolutionary Russian psychiatry had available only a few institutions for difficult and delinquent children and adolescents and a network of charitable orphanages and shelters for severely retarded and epileptic children.

Intensive work in the field of scientific psychiatry was undertaken after the October Revolution—despite the difficulties of the first years of revolution, civil war, and epidemics—at older university centers and at newly organized universities in outlying areas and the national republics. Investigative work continued to follow the traditional Russian psychiatric tendency toward solution of clinical problems, but also, in line with the requirements of the time, it became concerned with studying the scientific principles to be employed in reorganizing existing psychiatric institutions and planning new ones; the psychiatric consequences of the first imperialistic war and the civil war, of the epidemics of typhoid fever, of the prevalence of social diseases (tuberculosis, alcoholism, outbreaks of cocainism and other drug addictions during the civil war, etc.), and of other factors to be taken into account.

The theoretical basis common to all Soviet psychiatrists, the philosophy of dialectical materialism and, in biological science, I. P. Pavlov's physiological theory of higher nervous activity, united all research work and channeled it into a single methodological trend. It is thus understandable that Soviet psychiatrists had a not entirely consistent attitude toward the appearance in Soviet psychiatry of various types of idealistic, vulgarized, often inimical tendencies, which inevitably involved researchers in semantic tangles and fallacious constructs, ultimately creating a gap between theory and the pressing demands of public health. The physiological concepts traditional throughout the entire development of Russian clinical practice, which gave rise to I. M. Sechenov's physiological theory and then to I. P. Pavlov's theory of higher nervous activity, naturally entailed a tendency toward regarding the patient as a somatopsychic whole. This tendency was outstanding in all the theoretical pronouncements of Soviet clinicians and in everyday medical practice, and it was a natural outgrowth of the theoretical hypotheses of the leaders of Russian clinical practice during the first half of the nineteenth century. The clinical pronouncements of these luminaries are easily superimposed on the background of Sechenov-Pavlov physiological theory.

Pavlov's principles of protective inhibition, of the protective regimen followed at therapeutic institutions, and of the value of the physician's words as a therapeutic factor all provided a theoretical explanation of much that had long ago been deduced empirically in clinical practice. A new, "physiological" light was shed on the individual therapeutic approach to the patient, the psychotherapeutic "spirit," and the atmosphere of therapeutic institutions. A critical reexamination was then made of psychotherapeutic, psychohygienic and psychoprophylactic problems in order to eliminate everything foreign to the principles of Soviet psychiatry.

S. Freud's psychoanalytic method was unsuitable for the overwhelming majority of pre-Revolutionary Russian and Soviet psychiatrists. Individual adherents of Freudian psychoanalysis among Russian psychiatrists (N. A. Vyrubov, N. Ye. Osipov, O. B. Fel'tsman) attempted to popularize it in Russia during the period between 1910 and 1914; the journal *Psikhoterapiya* (Psychotherapy), which had a distinct psychoanalytic bias, was published in Moscow under the editorship of Vyrubov, with the close cooperation of a number of the most orthodox Viennese psychoanalysts. None of these attempts, however, had the desired success and, as before, Freudian psychoanalysis remained foreign to the majority of Russian psychiatrists. New attempts were made to popularize psychoanalysis in Soviet psychiatry after the October Revolution. During the 1920's, a whole series of volumes was published in the "Psychoanalytic Library" under the editorship of I. D. Yermakov, that were translations into Russian of the basic works of Freud and his closest followers. Attempts were made to relate Freudian psychoanalysis to Marxism (Yu. V. Kannabikh, V. A. Vnukov) as well as to understand communism from the Freudian standpoint (G. Yu. Malis). None of these attempts, however, met with any success and all went unnoticed by the majority of Soviet psychoanalysts. Modified, neo-Freudian forms were regarded by Soviet psychiatrists as blindly speculative, idealistic constructs having nothing in common with the philosophic methodology of dialectical materialism. In his very substantial monograph *Current Trends in Foreign Psychiatry and Their Ideological Origins*, V. M. Morozov quite correctly points out that the adherents of all these idealistic trends "usually consider man only as a biological entity whose behavior and feelings are determined by a few innate instincts, subconscious impulses, or primitive mechanical reactions to the environment." Indistinctly seen in the origins and causative factors of morbid neuropsychiatric conditions is an obscure biological force hidden in the depths of the personality. In his classic monograph *Psychopathological Symptomatology* (1933), P. B. Gannushkin, the head of the leading school of Soviet psychiatrists, and one who always maintained a very reserved attitude toward Freud's theories, felt it sufficient to relegate Freudian psychoanalysis to a footnote and pointed out that "the method by which Freud attempted to explain the genesis and symptomology of psychopathic conditions seems to us to be overly enigmatic, arbitrary, and indeterminate to be at all seriously applicable to such a vast and important problem."

The clinical-nosological trend and the tendency toward a patho-physiological view of mental disorders to a large extent protected Soviet psychiatry from fortuitous, methodologically foreign, and speculative elements. Discussions of theoretical problems in psychiatry and related biological disciplines, which took place over a period of years, uncovered the roots of the unwholesome, methodologically alien ideas and distortions that had crept into Soviet psychiatry and kept them from developing further. Thus, for example, the success of Soviet psychiatrists in the field of borderline conditions at the neuropsychiatric dispensaries and the sanitariums for neurological patients, and their direct guidance of extensive outpatient facilities for individual groups of workers, sponsored a tendency for individual physicians to accept extremely broad psychopathological criteria and to extrapolate uncritically the mechanisms of "major" psychiatric conditions to isolated neurotic and asthenic manifestations or to transient personality aberrations. Similar errors were committed in the psychiatry of early childhood.

This fact and the uncritical acceptance of Kretschmer's concept of the development of normal personality quirks into psychoses, a theory which erased the boundary between normal and pathological conditions, between normal personality traits and mental illness, led to an unjustified extension of the boundaries of such severe mental disorders as schizophrenia and to resultant severe consequences for persons thus classified as mentally ill. The necessary corrections were, however, made in all these overenthusiastic theories shortly after publication of a critical article by V. P. Osipov, one of the most eminent Soviet psychiatrists, which caused a heated debate at the Second All-Union Congress of Neuropathologists and Psychiatrists in 1936. A nearly analogous situation arose in another case: Extremely intense interest in the problem of the localization of psychic functions led to complex psychopathological theories based on the functional integrity of the body and brain and positing localization in quite restricted areas of the central nervous system. Such simplified concepts could only promote an uncritical extension of operative intervention in schizophrenia (by prefrontal leukotomy)—a technique employed in the Western nations—to the Soviet Union. Soon after checking the results of such operations, the Soviet psychiatric community raised the question of discontinuing this practice as antiphysiological and undoubtedly harmful.

Pedagogical interest in the psychopathology of children and adolescents was also severely criticized. In addition to the usual clinical-psychopathological study of symptoms of mental retardation undertaken at psychiatric clinics for children and adolescents, the study of academic failure and of pedagogic and social neglect had been limited by the simplified investigative techniques used for children and adolescents, which were elementary in character and so universal as to be described in all psychology texts, and by the offhand treatment of mentally healthy but congenitally retarded children, or defectives, who were transferred to auxiliary classes for the retarded. On the theoretical level practices of this type entailed the establishment of a new, independent discipline, *defectology,* lying somewhere between the natural and medical sciences and the pedagogical sciences. The founding of a separate discipline was naturally not justified in actuality and pointed up the total erroneousness of attributing the diverse factors underlying academic failure or pedagogic and social neglect solely to biological defects. All the pedological pitfalls discussed above were finally brought into the open at the First All-Union Conference on Human Behavior held in Moscow in 1930. Also, a number of problems of heredity and constitution were critically reexamined in general discussions held by scientific societies for neurologists and psychiatrists in Moscow, Leningrad, and other cities.

These and subsequent discussions overcame theoretically inadmissible and speculative tendencies, which were causing Soviet psychiatry to stray from the clinical-nosological path. This was to the advantage of the discipline, and it subsequently progressed unhampered to indubitable achievements in both theoretical and clinical psychiatry.

The persistent interest of pre-Revolutionary Russian psychiatrists in the problem of infectious psychoses is to a considerable extent attributable to the not infrequent epidemics of acute infectious diseases in Czarist Russia. During the Soviet era the successful conduct of epidemiological measures sharply reduced the incidence of acute infectious diseases, some of which (such as malaria) were almost entirely eliminated, and the interest of Soviet psychiatrists in them naturally decreased. However, during the first few years after the October Revolution, a period of economic upheaval, the shortage of foodstuffs and the pandemics of typhoid diseases attracted a great deal of attention by psychiatrists. Their interest was concentrated on elucidating the differences rather than the similarities among the mental disorders observed in the various forms of typhoid. However the clinical observations of psychiatrists later (in some cases during World War I, 1914–1917) came to be centered in the infectious-disease wards of general hospitals or in special hospitals for such diseases. Only here could the entire spectrum of psychopathological manifestations be observed in ordinary infectious diseases not exacerbated by complications in the central nervous system. Kraepelin pointed out the extraordinary value to psychiatry of observations made in infectious-disease wards. Such observations by Soviet psychiatrists made possible detection of unusual psychopathological nuances in ordinary cases of infectious diseases and descriptions of them as characteristic of a given type of infection. In some clinically unclear cases of infectious disease, correct evaluation of these peculiarities in the patient's mental state is of material aid in making a differential diagnosis of the basic affliction. This is particularly true in typhoid infections, where such differences are most pronounced.

The attention of Soviet psychiatrists was drawn both to the infectious-disease wards and to other departments of general medical hospitals. P. B. Gannushkin was always interested in and tried to make observations in somatic hospitals and was, until his death, a constant consultant at the S. P. Botkin Clinical Somatic Hospital. He was a strong supporter of the idea of organizing a psychiatric service and psychiatric wards at general hospitals. After his death in 1933, Gannushkin's views were put into practice, first at the Botkin Hospital and then at other medical hospitals. The clinical data gathered at somatic hospitals are of great interest to psychiatrists: They are the most promising and accessible materials for studying problems of corticovisceral relationship and the clinical relationship of mental and somatic phenomena under clinical conditions. As was seen from the foregoing discussion, the attempts of Russian and Soviet physicians in this direction, which began during the first half of the nineteenth century, were based on strictly clinical principles and physiological concepts of neuropsychiatric manifestations. These attempts by Soviet doctors cannot, however, be confused with the current American theory of psychosomatic medicine, which is based wholly and completely on modernized neo-Freudian depth-psychodynamic concepts and is essentially idealistic. These artificial constructs of the American psychosomatic theoreticians, foreign to the truly materialistic clinical-physiological trend in Soviet psychiatry, could not but repel Soviet psychiatrists and reduce their interest in this problem. Substantial progress was made in determining the relationship of mental and somatic phenomena by Soviet physiologists of Pavlov's school who used experimental data and data of the symptomatology of internal illness to study corticovisceral and viscerovisceral relationships.

In connection with the great importance which Soviet society has always attached to the protection of workers and to industrial medicine, Soviet psychiatrists devoted a great deal of attention also to intoxication psychoses and to mental disorders associated with occupational hazards, particularly at chemical enterprises. Some of these investigations were carried out in close cooperation with the V. A. Obukh Institute of Occupational Diseases in Moscow. The problem of chronic alcoholism and the treatment of alcoholics also occupied Soviet psychiatrists. Much attention was devoted to studying the initial signs of chronic alcohol poisoning of the nervous system and the systems of hangovers, while methods and drugs were sought for treating chronic alcoholism, particularly in connection with the development of conditioned-reflex-vomiting associations with the drinking of alcoholic beverages. The traditional interest of Russian and Soviet psychiatrists in the Korsakov syndrome has persisted down to the present, and their many investigations, both purely clinical and clinical-physiological, have occupied a rather prominent place in their scientific publications. Unfortunately, it has not been possible to establish anything conclusive about its physiological bases.

The problem of traumatic psychoses occupied Soviet psychiatrists throughout the entire period after the October Revolution and even during World War I. From the very beginning, the concept of traumatic neurosis drew criticism as somehow paradoxical, although more from psychiatrists than from neuropathologists. The mass of data on traumatization of the central nervous system compiled during World War II naturally occupied a central position in research work, after problems of schizophrenia. Of special interest and value in this series of investigations are studies devoted to higher nervous activity in the presence of traumatic injuries to the brain and subsequent dynamic observations made on patients with traumatic mental disorders. Pathomorphological data on cerebral traumas terminating in death at various stages of morbidity are also important. In addition to a whole series of interesting individual scientific conclusions, data on trauma gathered by dynamic observation quite clearly showed that mental disorders following cerebral trauma are not residual phenomena but manifestations of a general cerebral morbidity with a characteristic dynamic course through its various stages, and that often (when the outcome is unfavorable) these should be regarded as traumatic disease. Besides establishing definite pathophysiological mechanisms, the numerous investigations of higher nervous activity in the presence of cerebral traumas brought about a number of new, physiologically grounded therapeutic measures.

Soviet psychiatry has made an especially large number of studies of schizophrenia. These have concentrated on clarifying its symptomatology and limits and on studying its pathogenetic mechanisms, the purpose being to confirm its nosological independence and to differentiate it from schizophrenia-like psychopathological conditions of differing nosological character. The expansion and concentration of research in this area and the search for the etiological and ophrenic conditions enabled the overwhelming majority of Soviet psychiatrists to take firm clinical positions and to recognize the nosological independence of schizophrenia as a processual disease. The extreme frequency with which diagnoses of "mild schizophrenia" were given played a positive role, since it properly attracted the attention of psychiatrists to the undoubted existence of cases of schizophrenia with a not very distinct processual symptomatology and a comparatively favorable course. This indubitable clinical fact, which was also noted in other branches of medicine, permitted a closer approach to the problem of the course and outcome of schizophrenia and the role played in this disease by the compensatory reserves of the nervous system; all these data also made possible reexamination of the validity of the almost universally accepted German hypothesis regarding the hereditary nature of schizophrenia.

A great deal of progress was also made as a result of the precise elaboration of the phenomenology of schizophrenia. In addition, Soviet psychiatrists devoted much attention to examining various aspects of disruptions of higher nervous activity in schizophrenia; there were numerous virological, immunobiological, and especially biochemical studies of the pathogenesis of the disease; and the problem of disruptions of cerebral electrical activity stimulated further interest. A broad range of purposeful, intensive, and successful research (both clinical-psychopathological and biological) studied the regularities in the course of syndrome sequence of the various stages of schizophrenia and its specific forms.

At the same time, intensive research was conducted at ordinary clinical institutions, psychiatric hospitals, dispensaries, and semiclinics. This work was directed primarily at clinical verification of old drugs and discovery of new, more effective ones for use in various types of psychoses; schizophrenia was naturally of primary interest.

Important investigations were conducted to elucidate the physiological bases of various types of hallucinatory phenomena and detrimental experiences (further developing I. P. Pavlov's theories on these problems) and compulsive phenomena. Soviet psychiatrists and physiologists also researched the physiological mechanisms underlying psychopathological manifestations in other nosological forms and clinically dominant syndromes.

Investigation in the field of "minor psychiatry" and borderline conditions was promoted by the fact that the most authoritative of the Soviet clinical psychiatrists, P. B. Gannushkin, a leading student of the classicists of Soviet psychiatry, S. S. Korsakov and V. P. Serbskiy, undertook his first clinical work in this area at the beginning of the century under the supervision of and in collaboration with his old colleague F. A. Sukhanov. The directions taken by their research subsequently diverged. While Sukhanov attempted to verify the possibility for pathological character traits to be psychopathologically intensified into corresponding forms of psychosis—a path taken considerably later in Germany by Kretschmer, which ultimately led him to his aforementioned theory unacceptable to Soviet psychiatrists—Gannushkin felt it impossible to stray from strictly clinical facts. This field of Soviet psychiatry is now wholly associated with Gannushkin. His classic, posthumously published monograph *Psychopathological Symptomatology* (1933) reflects his thirty years of observation and theorizing in this area of clinical practice. His understanding of psychopathic conditions rested entirely on a sober evaluation of actual clinical data and lacked the often-encountered, simplified tendency to attribute all the diversity of specific data to the constitutional-hereditary roots of personality or to the action of fortuitous detrimental environmental factors. The former view completely ignores the significance of the external, primarily social environment in forming personality, whereas the latter overlooks the role of the biological bases of personality traits. As is well known, the majority of researchers, both Soviet and foreign, have adopted one of these two equally one-sided positions.

In taking into account the various aspects of the symptomatology of psychopathic conditions (static, dynamic, and phaselike), Gannushkin came very close to a physiological view of his clinical data and essentially paved the way for subsequent special physiological investigations in this area. He gave a clear account of the complications and difficulties which arise in any psychopathological investigation, and he emphasized that in his systematics of psychopathic conditions he proceeded solely from specific clinical data and did not permit himself to go farther than they warranted. At this stage of our knowledge we can consequently speak only of an empirical systematics of psychopathology, its statics and dynamics.

The entire force and significance of Gannushkin's theory of psychopathic conditions lies in his scientific strictness and thoroughness as a leading clinician and in his fear of premature, unverified, and speculative conclusions and generalizations. The majority of the work of other Soviet psychiatrists in this field is at the same level. Attempts to distinguish special types of psychopathic conditions based solely on social factors were unsuccessful both methodologically and clinically and have received no support in the literature. Unfortunately, no sufficiently convincing results have yet been yielded by attempts to construct a classification of psychopathic conditions on the basis of Pavlov's theory of nervous-system types. In recent years O. V. Kerbikov and his colleagues have tried to expand Gannushkin's theory of psychopathic dynamics by including transient psychopathoid conditions (which in some cases subsequently acquire a stable character), whose development is based solely on unfavorably complicated living conditions and unendurable situations, especially during the early stages of the formation of the conscious personality.

Specialists in mental illnesses of childhood and adolescence have introduced much of value into general Soviet psychiatry. In addition to working out the symptomatology of psychoses in these age groups, establishing precise differential-diagnostic criteria, and determining the symptomatological differences between childhood and adult illnesses, child psychiatrists furnished a great deal of support for the development of "adult psychiatry." They also contributed greatly to the clarification of the role of a number of other factors in the development of mental illnesses and abnormalities during the introuterine development of the fetus, delivery, and the postnatal period. Further, they increased our understanding of the functional development of the endocrine system and juvenile "brain infections" and other abnormalities to which children are subject but which are often overlooked in collecting anamnestic data at a later time and thus are not given sufficient consideration.

The scientific output of psychiatrists increased substantially during the Soviet era in comparison with that of the pre-Revolutionary years. This is attributable to the fact that the number of psychiatric workers rose considerably with the organization of special psychoneurological research institutes and medical schools with independent departments of psychiatry in many cities; and the instructors in these departments of psychiatry conducted a great deal of research in addition to their teaching, in keeping with the long-standing traditions of Russian universities. Research also attracted many physicians employed at psychiatric hospitals and dispensaries. The changes which took place in the publication of the results of scientific investigations are understandable if one takes into account the fact that the transactions of numerous scientific and scientific-practical conferences, meetings, and congresses had to be published. The situation gradually developed to the point that the majority of scientific papers appeared in collections, which were brought out as the scientific-research institutes and departments of psychiatry of medical institutes amassed material, as well as in special collections of scientific reports on the work of general and local psychiatric (sometimes in conjunction with neuropathological) congresses and meetings. At the same time, the number of journals of psychiatry and neuropathology was gradually reduced, so that there now remains only one, the oldest psychiatric periodical, first published in 1901, the S. S. Korsakov Journal of Neuropathology and Psychiatry. The advantage of this publication system for the majority of scientific papers lies, among other things, in the fact that it attracts local medical personnel to research and permits expansion and guidance of local investigative work. All this is of especially great importance for psychiatrists in the outlying republics, which were the most neglected in this respect in Czarist Russia.

The following facts also show the intensity of the research being conducted in the Soviet Union in comparison with that of the pre-Revolutionary period. During the entire era of the development of scientific psychiatry in Russia, i.e., from the second half of the nineteenth century until the Revolution in 1917, scientific and scientific-organizational problems and narrower problems of psychiatric practice were considered at four congresses of Russian psychiatrists and at the Congress of the Association of Russian Psychiatrists and Neuropathologists (in 1887, 1904, 1909, and 1911), as well as at the Sections for Nervous and Mental Illnesses of five Congresses of Russian Physicians in Memory of N. I. Pirogov (between 1891 and 1904). After the February and October Revolutions of 1917 four All-Russian Conferences of Psychiatrists and Neuropathologists were held (in 1917, another in 1917, 1919, and 1923), as were four All-Union Congresses of Neuropathologists and Psychiatrists that involved a series of parallel sectional meetings on child psychiatry, forensic psychiatry, military psychiatry, and the function of the dissector in psychiatric clinics and hospitals (in 1917, 1936, 1948, and 1963). There were also many local psychiatric conferences, both in the central regions of the nation and in the various republics and territories. The majority of these local sectional meetings, especially those in the capitals of republics and the seats of territories, were well attended by participants from the entire Soviet Union. For example, the conference commemorating the fiftieth anniversary of the founding of the Psychiatric Clinic of Moscow University at Devichiy Polye attracted psychiatrists from almost all the regions and republics, and the scientific conference held at the same psychiatric clinic by the First

Moscow Medical Institute in 1951 to commemorate the one-hundredth anniversary of the birth of S. S. Korsakov was no less well attended and saw many scientific papers presented. The same was true of the Combined Session of the Presidium of the U.S.S.R. Academy of Medical Sciences and the Executive Board of the All-Union Scientific Society of Neuropathologists and Psychiatrists in 1951, and of the psychoneurological congresses in the Ukraine, the Central Asiatic Republics (in Tashkent), the Baltic republics (in Riga), Armenia, Georgia, Azerbaydzhan, Moldavia, etc.

The Scientific Psychiatric Association of the Soviet Union comprises the All-Union Scientific Society of Neuropathologists and Psychiatrists and the corresponding scientific societies of neuropathologists and psychiatrists in the Union republics, which are affiliates of the All-Union Scientific Society. In turn the Psychiatric Association of the Russian Federation includes the All-Russian Scientific Society of Neuropathologists and Psychiatrists and its affiliates in the capitals of the autonomous republics and in the seats of the regions and territories. Each year, at an expanded plenary session, the Executive Board of the All-Union Society summarizes the work done during the year in the Report of the Chairman, which is followed by election of a new Executive Board. The plenary session of the Executive Board of the Society is usually coordinated with some scientific conference or meeting of interest to all psychiatrists in the Soviet Union.

Instruction in psychiatry is obligatory in all faculties of the medical institutes, but few hours are devoted to lectures and practical work in this area in the sanitation-hygiene faculty. Psychiatry, as the clinical discipline which culminates the development of a profoundly synthetic clinical way of thought in medical students, is taught in the last years of medical school, after the other clinical disciplines. The instructor in psychiatry thus has the very weighty task of using his clinical material to show the complex of causal factors producing the clinical pattern of illness in each patient and the importance of an integral view of the complicated individual psychosomatic organization of the patient. In former years, when the teaching load on medical faculties was not so heavy, psychiatry was taught in the last three semesters (of a five-year program). During the second semester of the fourth year, the students were familiarized with the history of psychiatry, the general principles of the organization of psychiatric aid, the place of psychiatry in medicine, etc., and they made a thorough study of the symptoms and psychopathological syndromes most frequently encountered in the clinic in mental illnesses. The final two semesters (the fifth year) were devoted to hospital work, to the study of the individual forms of psychosis and related problems of general clinical methodology, to acquisition of an integral view of the patient and a proper bedside manner, etc. As a result of the load on teaching programs in medical institutes, the number of hours now devoted to the teaching of psychiatry is greatly curtailed, not corresponding to the demands on or the value of psychiatry in general medical practice. The therapeutic faculties devote thirty-six hours of lectures and fifty hours of practical work to psychiatry, the sanitation-hygiene faculties eighteen and thirty-six hours respectively. The specialized pediatric faculties devote a few hours as well.

The authors of Soviet textbooks on psychiatry have attempted to compensate for the lack of time devoted to teaching psychiatry, taking this circumstance into account and, as far as possible, improving both their manner of presentation and the character and sequence of their material. The most informative of these texts are the often-reissued *Textbook of Psychiatry* by V. A. Gilyarovskiy and M. O. Guervich and the *Handbook of Psychiatry* by O. F. Kerbikov, N. I. Ozeretskiy, Ye. A. Popov, and A. V. Snezhnevskiy. The latter is based wholly on Pavlov's theory of the physiology of higher nervous activity. The psychiatric community also generally approves O. V. Kerbikov's *Clinical Lectures on Psychiatry,* A. S. Chistovich's *Manual of Psychiatry,* I. F. Sluchevskiy's *Psychiatry,* and G. Ye. Sukharev's *Lectures on Child Psychiatry.* The classical texts on general psychiatry are still those by S. S. Korsakov and V. P. Osipov; that on psychopathic conditions is P. B. Gannushkin's *Psychopathological Symptomatology.*

The large network of medical schools and scientific research psychiatric institutes in the Soviet Union necessitates serious attention to the problem of preparing scientific personnel and instructors in this field. The number of doctors employed at therapeutic institutions and simultaneously conducting fruitful research has increased considerably. The training of highly skilled specialists for hospitals and for the network of outpatient institutions is a major task. Because psychiatric aid is being provided for the populace by decentralization of clinics and expansion of the network of outpatient dispensaries and clinics, the network of psychiatric institutions requires more and more new medical personnel. After they have completed medical school, young physicians are given specialized training in psychiatry by institutes for residents at the psychiatric clinics of medical or scientific-research institutes and at the majority of municipal and regional psychiatric hospitals. The term of residence is two years. On completion of their residency the young specialists either remain at the local psychiatric institutions where they received specialized training or are sent by the Ministry of Public Health or the Region Public Health Services to therapeutic institutions in greater need of medical personnel; understandably these are for the most part in outlying areas. There is a system of graduate study for training scientific workers from among doctors who have completed their specialization in psychiatry. Graduate students in clinical psychiatry are selected from among young specialists with the greatest aptitude for research who have worked at least two years in therapeutic institutions of their specialty and have successfully passed entrance examinations in their basic specialty, in related disciplines, and in the principles of dialectic materialism. The maximum age for admission to graduate study is thirty-five years. The program for training of graduate students provides for completion of three years of study and successful defense of a dissertation at the academic level of Candidate of Medical Sciences. On completion of their studies the young research workers are assigned to permanent jobs, usually at one of the scientific-research institutes of psychiatry or at the departments of psychiatry of medical institutes. The assignment is at the discretion of the All-Union or Republic Ministries of Public Health.

In addition to the extensive network of medical institutes, there are also Institutes for the Advanced Training of Physicians in a number of large cities and the capitals of the Union republics. Practicing physicians, including psychiatrists, are sent to these institutes in a definite sequence and at set intervals for advanced training in their specialty. Instruction is carried out in accordance with a strict program centered on problems of the symptomatology and diagnosis of mental illnesses and familiarization with modern methods for treating the mentally ill. In some cases, courses have been set up for requalification from one clinical specialty to another and for primary specialization in psychiatry. Individual short-term courses in the most pressing problems of psychiatry are organized sporadically.

CHAPTER THREE

Psychotherapy in the German Democratic Republic

BY
DR. D. MÜLLER-HEGEMANN

HISTORY

PSYCHIATRY IN THE GERMAN DEMOCRATIC REPUBLIC (GDR) did not develop in any different manner from that in West Germany until 1945. The centers of scientific and practical work were six university clinics: Berlin, Leipzig, Jena, Halle, Rostock, and Greifswals, where psychiatrists of international rank were active.* Some municipal clinics also earned substantial distinction. Most notable was the clinic in Dresden, where Ganser described the syndrome of strong hysterical manifestations accompanied by pseudo dementia. In addition, there were a number of well-known psychiatric institutions, for example, Alt Scherbitz, near Leipzig. Alt Scherbitz was founded on the expansive grounds of an old estate, and patients were given extensive freedom in connection with a full program of work therapy. The institution is best known for its pioneer activity at the end of the nineteenth century in this program.

---

* In Berlin, W. Griesinger, C. Westphal, and K. Bonthoeffer; in Leipzig, P. Glechsig and P. Schroder; in Jena, O. Binswanger and H. Berger; in Halle, C. Wernicke and G. Anton; and in Rostock, O. Bumke and K. Kleist.

The clinical institutions of Berlin occupied a dominant position through the decades. W. Griesinger in the late nineteenth century founded the Psychiatric and Neurological Clinic of the University at the Berlin Charity Hosiptal, a connection between psychiatry and neurology which became the prototype in all parts of Germany. By grouping mental illness with nervous disease Griesinger placed the treatment of the mentally ill on a par with physical illnesses. This had the effect of discouraging the moralistic psychiatry of Heinroth and Ideler, who held some mental illnesses to be the result of sin.

Griesinger sought at the same time a "psychiatric attitude," i.e., maximum understanding and avoidance of compulsory methods toward even aggravated and aggressive patients. He valued the importance of psychic influences in the pathogenesis of mental illnesses but recognized the need to wait for the time "when the questions of the connection of the content of human psychic life with its form become physiological rather than metaphysical 'problems.'" He can be considered a forerunner of I. P. Pavlov, since he interpreted the psychic phenomena as originating in reflexes.

Under the influence of Griesinger it became customary in Germany to train in psychiatry as well as in neurology. This circumstance, however, did not exclude the influence of the leading specialists in neurology, like Oppenheim and Cassirer in Berlin and V. Strumpell in Leipzig, or the specialists in brain research and neuropathology, like O. Vogt and H. Spatz in Berlin and P. Flechsig and R. A. Pfeifer in Leipzig.

The years 1933–1945, i.e., the time of the fascist dictatorship, brought greater trouble for neurological psychiatry than for any other special medical discipline. Unscientific, antihuman theories and practices were declared as official doctrine in the "laws of July 14, 1933, to prevent growth of hereditary diseases," according to which tens of thousands of psychiatric patients, especially those with mild forms of schizophrenia, manic-depressive illness, oligophrenia, etc., were forced to undergo mass sterilization. These laws are to be distinguished, however, from the absolutely criminal "euthanasia" methods in the second half of the fascist dictatorship, by which many thousands were systematically killed as incurable. These mass murders were not based on legal grounds; they were due to a secret order of the Führer.

Although a number of German psychiatrists were ordered to participate in these crimes by the authorities—for which they were held responsible at the end of the war—the majority of psychiatrists remained faithful to the humanitarian principles of medicine. They did their utmost to protect the patients entrusted to them from the destructive clutches of the fascist state organization.

After the war ended in 1945, every German psychiatrist had to re-examine his theoretical and practical views in psychiatry. Eugenics as represented in Germany until 1945—as the social-Darwinist propagation of a superbreed—publicly and fully appeared as unscientific. It cannot be overlooked that a one-time competent German psychiatrist, A. Hoche, proposed the killing of incurably sick or defective people back in 1920 in a paper entitled "The Right to Destroy Worthless Life." Hoche bolstered his argument with a theory of a predetermined endogeny in the etiology of schizophrenia, manic-depressive illness, and other widespread illnesses. The leading advocate of these theories of compulsory sterilization was E. Rudkin. In the early post-war years there was a general arousal of conscience concerning the important traditions of psychiatry, as represented by the names of W. Griesinger, C. Wernicke, E. Kraepelin, R. Gaupp, K. Bonhoffer.

Thereafter there was a sharp division between the German Federal Republic (western) and the German Democratic Republic (eastern) regarding the American-developed "dynamic psychiatry." Psychiatry advanced in different directions in the split Germany, with psychoanalysis, psychosomatic medicine, and existential analysis in the West and the teaching of Pavlov in the East. The majority of active psychiatrists in both the East and the West carefully followed a conservative position. And despite the different new directions taken by psychiatry in East and West Germany, there was manifested a common factor, which was rejection of the previously dominant German teaching of endogeny. Here psychiatrists in all of Germany continued their relationnships, so that a basis was established for theoretical discussions.

ORGANIZATIONAL ADVANCES IN PSYCHIATRY

Some well-established medical schools have seen the following developments since the war:

The University of Berlin's Neurological Clinic (Charity) was directed by R. Thiele after the war and has been under the direction of K. Leonhard since 1954. These two internationally respected neurological psychiatrists have restored the clinic to its previous eminence through their scientific studies of important problems in neurology, psychiatry, and psychopathology. The organizational development of the clinic also has advanced substantially, with special departments for psychiatry and neurology, neuroradiology, and child psychiatry. In addition, new divisions of psychotherapy, electroencephalography, neuropathology, and forensic psychiatry were set up, and distinguished research and practice has resulted.

The Leipzig Clinic, which was totally destroyed in 1943, was reestablished by the famous brain researcher R. A. Pfeifer after the war. D. Müller-Hegemann directed the clinic from 1951 to 1964. The old departments for psychiatry, neurology, and child neuropsychiatry were augmented during the past twelve years by departments for psychotherapy, neuroradiology, electroencephalography, and clinical neurophysiology. The most scientific work was performed in psychotherapy, social psychiatry, child neuropsychiatry, research in cerebral-cortical disturbance, and the application of the principal teachings of Pavlov. R. A. Pfeifer also established a brain-research institute in Leipzig shortly after the war, which has been headed by W. Wunscher since 1957. Recently the morphological-research section at the institute was expanded into a neurochemical department.

The neurological clinic in Jena was named "Hans Berger Clinic" as a tribute to the intensive research done by Berger in discovering and developing electroencephalography. After the war the director of the clinic was R. Lemke, later followed by V. Keyserlingk. Lemke dealt with problems of neuroradiology and the artistic forms of expression in psychopathology, and V. Keyserlingk dealt with alcoholism and social problems.

The clinic in Halle, under the direction of K. Ponitz, regained its previous distinguished place after the war. It is now headed by H. Rennert, a prominent member of the Société Internationale de Psychopathologie de l'Expression. The Rostock clinic was the first to set up independent chairs in psychiatry and child psychiatry. The clinic in Sayk has specialized in alcohol studies and neurology. H. Schwarz, who directs the clinic in Greifswald, has contributed many important studies to addiction, psychopharmacology, and clinical psychiatry.

The recently established (1955–1956) medical academies in Dresden, Erfurt, and Magdeburg have in the short time of their existence achieved about the same status as the other university clinics and are similarly centers of academic training and research. Finally, there is the newly created (1961) Chair of Psychiatry and Neurology at the German Academy for Postgraduate Medicine in Berlin, which is under the direction of D. Müller-Hegemann. This new academic establishment will lead to valuable postgraduate training and will undoubtedly attract medical specialists to the GDR for additional schooling.

The total number of psychiatric beds, largely in psychiatric hospitals, in the GDR amounted to 30,843 for a population of 17,135,867 in 1963.* The big hospitals have their own neuropathological, x-ray, and electroencephalography departments. Lately, many psychiatric hospitals have developed new forms of patient care, especially day care. An example is the Wuhlgarten municipal hospital in Berlin with a day-care unit for forty patients. There is also a night center for patients who work during the day. Work therapy is prescribed for most patients. The principles of the open-door system, and sociotherapy, combined with medication, injections, and insulin therapy, are widely used.

Ambulant care is likewise to be found in state polyclinics and private state medical practice. There are extensive psychiatric consulting offices which engage in aftercare as well for patients with continuous psychoses and for difficult psychopaths and alcoholics.

Until a few years ago there was a great shortage of physicians. Recently, there has been a high-grade increase of graduates in the medical faculties and academies. The number of psychiatric neurological specialists in the next five to six years will rise to 1,000, according to the analyses and proposals of the Association for Psychiatry and Neurology in the German Democratic Republic, which is directed by K. Leonhard.

Both this society and the Society for Medical Psychotherapy, founded a few years ago by D. Müller-Hegemann, regularly hold large congresses and symposia with international participation. The affiliated six regional societies of the Psychiatric-Neurological Society (in Berlin, Leipzig, Jena, Halle, Rostock-Greifswald, and Dresden) also hold annual conferences and meetings which provide opportunities of communication on the progress of scientific work. It is a regular practice to invite West German psychiatrists to the central and regional programs. The monthly journal "Psychiatrie, Neurologie und Med. Psychologie," under the editorship of D. Müller-Hegemann, is the organ of these societies.

THE POSITION OF SCIENTIFIC DISCUSSION

Problems of Psychoses

The discussion of problems of psychoses has been undertaken by K. Leonhard, whose papers on endogenous psychoses are internationally known. In a significant monograph he distinguishes four main groups:

* Statistical Yearbook of the GDR, 1963.

1. Phasic psychoses
2. Cyclic psychoses
3. Unsystematic schizophrenia
4. Systematic schizophrenia

The phasic psychoses are subdivided into (*a*) manic-depressive illness, (*b*) pure melancholy and mania, and (*c*) pure depressions and pure euphoria; the cyclic psychoses into (*a*) anxiety-good-fortune psychoses, (*b*) disturbance-triggered entanglement (confusion), and (*c*) hyperkinetic-akinetic spontaneous psychoses. With regard to both schizophrenic main groups he differentiates many subgroups as well as the systematic schizophrenia: (*a*) simple systematic schizophrenia, and (*b*) combined systematic schizophrenia, primarily catatonic forms which are again subdivided as:

1. Parakinetic
2. Affective
3. Proskinetic
4. Negativist
5. Speech (expressive) ready
6. Speech-supporting catatonic forms

It may lead us too far afield to cover here all the different forms he mentions, which total thirty-eight in number. It is important to know that Leonhard's conclusions are based on extensive clinical experience. He cites 526 phasic psychoses and 324 cases of schizophrenia as "demonstrated cases" of his research.

Mention should be made of Leonhard's work in collaboration with V. Trostorff. Here it became clear that he followed Kraepelin's *Verlaufspsychiatrie* conception in his description of a curable (manic-depressive illness) and an incurable (schizophrenic) group of endogenetic psychoses. However he departs from Kraepelin (whose methods of diagnosis he considered limited in differentiation) in his proposal of the numerous different forms of psychoses mentioned above. Leonhard's conception of endogenous psychoses did not stand unopposed, even in the German Democratic Republic. At the 1963 Congress for Psychiatry, in Dresden, H. Rennert and Kesker (Heidelberg, West Germany) both made critical remarks.[21] Rennert noted that the empirical bases can be accepted at the earliest time (*ebesten*) if it is considered a syndrome and not a disease.

At the same time, Rennert argued against the traditional Kraepelinian division of two endogenous psychoses and supported the earlier nineteenth-century concept of an endogenous "unified psychosis." Rennert stands alone in this view in the German Democratic Republic. It is generally held that the Kraepelinian distinction between "manic-depressive" illness and schizophrenia is a medical and historical advance to be renounced only when positive new knowledge is available.

Müller-Hegemann expresses the majority view in his textbook "Neurology and Psychiatry."[14] Here he points to basic differences between both illnesses, including not only the duration of symptoms but also the premorbid (especially the emotional) characteristics of the patients. The subdivisions of endogenous psychoses are discussed in the book "Psychoses Without Probed Causes." The emphasis on endogenesis is indicative of our current lack of knowledge of definite criteria of neurological, neuropathological, and neurochemical factors.

Hence there are a few subgroups such as the schizophrenic, paranoic-hallucinatory, catatonic, hebephrenic, and paraphrenic forms, as well as schizophrenia simplex. The incidence of atypical psychoses of this sort is not challenged; the many sickness forms (especially involutional psychoses) are conditioned in large number and take hold as reactive (participating strongly in psychogenic periods). The share of last-named psychoses in the sum total of psychoses is regarded as considerable.

The role of Kraepelin is confirmed in this connection. He recognized not only endogenous or other organically based psychoses, but also reactive psychoses as well. Thus emotional disorders may arise from hearing difficulties and hamper the "contact" between people. In an article Müller-Hegemann describes numerous reactive psychoses in the hard-of-hearing developing from social isolation, distressing migration circumstances, or difficult conflict situations.[1] At the same time he points out that the necessary expansion of the science of psychiatry through the recognition of reactive psychoses and, hence, also the need for psychotherapeutic practice on psychotic patients do not provide any basis for the rejection of, in its essential characteristics, Kraepelin's teaching.

Other authoritative psychiatrists of the GDR, for example, E. Lange (Dresden), have referred to the significance of reactive psychoses. The majority of GDR psychiatrists, however, still adhere to a conservative principle which on the whole is based on Kraepelin's teaching without sufficiently considering its progressive elements. Thus, one often finds a marked emphasis on the endogenous factor—in regard to organic nonsubstantiated psychoses as well as to psychopathy and neurosis phenomena.

Problems of the Teaching of Neuroses and Psychotherapy

In the field of the teaching of neuroses and psychotherapy, as well as in other fields of psychiatry, there have developed in the past twenty years greater contrasts between the western and eastern parts of Germany. Although no pure "Pavlovian" trend has prevailed in the GDR, a clinically substantiated, empirical, Pavlov-oriented psychotherapy is dominant at present. However, the representative and applied methods are far from uniform; there are many differences, for instance, between Leonhard's "individual therapy," employed in Berlin, and Müller-Hegemann's "rational psychotherapy" as practiced in Dresden. In contrast to this, the deep psychological, existential-analytical, existentialist, and similar trends have found very few adherents. This profound contrast with the concepts adhered to in West Germany is not ultimately the result of theoretical discussions. Rather, Professor A. Mette* is largely responsible for the dominant trends in the GDR. For many years before assuming his present position, he was active as a psychoanalyst. He devoted far-reaching investigations into the theoretical principles of psychoanalysis and deep psychological teaching connected with it, and in the course of his studies he changed his previous approach. One can refer to his biography, "Sigmund Freud,"[10] in which he shows how Freud's rejection of the scientific and clinical scope of experience and his one-sided turning to the psychic phenomena of patients, especially their dreams and instinct experiences, has resulted in an overgrowth of the weeds of speculation. At the same time Mette points out the biologistic and mechanistic features in Freud's and his followers' teachings, which find in the thought process an expression of the instinct energetics. Mette leans toward Pavlov's teaching, which has an incomparably stronger empirical basis in neurophysiology than Freud's and which, through the discovery of conditional-reflex laws, involves also the psychic phenomena.

Opinions essentially similar to Mette's are held by Müller-Hegemann.[16] Müller-Hegemann's system also involves the regular hospital and ambulatory use of autogenous training, which use has spread far beyond the German frontiers. This is interpreted as training of the cerebral hemispheres—creating new conditioned-reflex links which induce tranquilization and normalize vasovegetative functions. Additional extensive use is made of external suggestive effects (with recorded tapes), including

* Director of the Institute of History of Medicine and Technical Director at the Humboldt University of Berlin.

hypnosis to obtain tranquilization and therapeutic sleep during the first stage of therapy. In the next stage, occupational therapy, gymnastics, musical therapy, and single and group sessions are primarily stressed. For severe neuroses, his method also involves continued long-term psychotherapeutic sessions to obtain deep and lasting redirections in the patient. Freud's "transference" concept is rejected as empirically unfounded; so is his extreme opinion that the "unconscious" as an "independent realm" plays a dominant role in mental life. However, unconscious processes are assigned great importance in neurotic disturbances.

According to Müller-Hegemann, psychotherapy is highly important not only in the treatment of neuroses but also as complementary treatment in psychoses and organic disease. Therefore, his textbook "Neurology and Psychiatry"[14] has a special psychotherapeutic section for each important chapter. Optimal psychotherapy is viewed as a synthesis of symptomatic, in part conditioned-reflex therapy and of causal, highly patient-specific therapy, with reference to case histories.[13]

Leonhard calls his method of treatment "individual therapy."[7] In explaining the three main forms (hysterical, anankastic, and sensohypochondriacal neuroses), he says that hysterical neuroses differ from other neuroses by a basic "desire for illness." A severe phobia will always reveal an anankastic constitution. The personalities of hysteric and compulsive patients are basically different. The latter are characterized by an over-conscientious way of life and are frequently tormented by their illness. With respect to hypochondria, he distinguishes between "sensohypochondriacal evolution," accompanied by subjective illusive sensations, and "ideohypochondriacal" disturbances, consisting in pathologic ideation, apprehension, or convictions. This is essentially a phobia referring to the patient's own body.

Therapeutic measures are highly specific for the respective forms. Before going into the particulars, we would describe the overall method as follows: therapeutic exercises are prescribed in detail and to an extent such as to occupy the greater part of the day. Persistence in their execution is considered important for achieving a "change" in the patient's habits. If necessary, long psychotherapeutic sessions are conducted, aimed mainly at convincing the patient of the need for minute execution of the program prescribed. In contrast to Müller-Hegemann, Leonhard restricts hospital therapy to this kind; he rejects simultaneous chemotherapy. Patients who require medication are not subjected to "individual therapy" nor to autogenous training and hypnosis. There is, however, agreement between the two on the importance of occupational and work therapy and therapeutic sports activities or gymnastics. Leonhard prescribes gradually increasing muscular stress for his patients, up to several hours daily for sports. The following details merit attention: in hysterical neurotics he stresses intensive therapy aimed at a change in habits, during which constant appeal must be made to the patient's own willpower. The opposite is required for the compulsive, tormented individual who must be assured that during the long conversations his therapist has become acquainted with his profound sense of responsibility and his conscientious personality. He would be rightly offended if his will to get well were doubted. In his case, active training for a change of habits is important also for daily life. If his compulsion makes it impossible for him to cross a bridge, he will accomplish it if the physician in whom he confides accompanies him there while diverting his attention with conversation and, if need be, pushes him gently across the bridge. In such cases, it takes sensitivity and time for persistent continuation of therapeutic measures. Sensohypochondriacs require similar procedures of diversion and a change of habits.

With respect to other important disturbances, e.g., stuttering, he considers it necessary to induce "normal automatization"; he makes the patient speak up to four hours a day, reading long texts until he is, as it were, unable to continue stuttering. Similarly, he recommends that patients with occupational neuroses be persuaded to persist at their work until the disturbance disappears. (Someone with writer's cramp is urged to continue writing until the symptoms disappear.)

In anorexia nervosa Leonhard recommends persistent feeding of the patients or asking them to feed themselves on the assurance that they are able to eat and would thus gain several pounds a month. If nausea develops, the patients are at once diverted to keep them from vomiting. Due to his extraordinary persistence, Leonhard has been able to interrupt the vicious circle in a surprisingly large number of these and other disturbances. For neurotic tics he talks about "breaking" this "automatism," which will give him a good basis for the subsequent psychotherapeutic treatment combined with therapeutic gymnastics and occupational therapy.

In the majority of mental clinics and the large psychiatric hospitals of the German Democratic Republic, psychotherapy is conducted methodically by means of autogenous training, single and group sessions, therapeutic gymnastics and occupational therapy. Several hospitals have special psychotherapeutic departments (Görden, Uchtspringe, Stadtroda) where therapeutic sleep similar to that in the Leipzig clinic is induced, i.e., by means of sleep-inducing tape-recorded suggestions using minimally required doses of hypnotics.

Methods of psychiatric treatment developed by H. Simon in Gütersloh (Westphalia) about forty years ago may also be considered psychotherapy.[23] These center around carefully graded work therapy aimed at leading the psychotic or retarded patient from simple to increasingly differentiated activities and are combined with milieu therapy featuring comfortably furnished rooms and the grouping of patients such as to favor interpersonal beneficial effects and the common execution of internal tasks (preparation of meals, food service, cleaning, etc.). The promotion of cultural activities assumes a similarly important role with regularly conducted group games, reading of books, singing, theater performances, etc. Therapeutic sports or gymnastics at scheduled intervals are just as important. In reference to H. Simon, the expression "collective psychotherapy" has often been used, particularly since exceptional individual psychotherapy is only possible in the psychiatric hospitals with their large number of patients. Schizophrenic patients, especially, responded with excellent results to this method. In the large mental hospitals of the GDR, Simon's method has remained, with slight modifications, the model for psychotherapy, and it is felt that without it no modern chemotherapy or shock therapy can exert its full effect.

Except for the therapy of psychoses, there is close collaboration in the field of psychotherapy between leading internists and neuropsychiatrists in the GDR. H. Kleinsorge (now at Schwerin) did much fruitful work as Director of the Medical University Polyclinic at Jena; so has his successor, G. Klumbies.[4] Their method involves a highly differentiated autogenous training, similarly specific therapeutic hypnosis, group therapy, and individual sessions.

A collection of readings[20] published in 1959 affords insight into the close collaboration that exists in the GDR between neuropsychiatrists, internists, and other specialists. The Leipzig group* reported on problems of neuroses in neuropsychiatry; the Jena circle† on problems of neuroses relating to internal disease (heart and circulatory diseases, digestive disturbances, endocrine and metabolic diseases, the various vegetative symptoms, etc.). Specialists in tuberculosis, gynecology, and dermatology‡ made contributions on the importance of neuroses in these fields. There was agreement from all branches of medicine on the important role of neurotic manifestations in many patients. When there are severe neurotic manifestations, it is the neuropsychiatrist's duty to establish the differential

* D. Müller-Hegemann, H. Wendt, B. Schwartz, and C. Wieck.
† H. Kleinsorge, G. Lumbies, G. Dornbusch, and G. Bolland.
‡ H. Marchand, N. Aresin, and P. G. Heese, respectively.

diagnosis between psychopathy and psychosis. If neurotic disturbances involve organs outside the nervous system, the respective specialist is called upon for diagnostic elucidation and to carry out independent psychotherapy if he has the necessary experience. The Society for Medical Psychotherapy recommends the creation of a "Specialist for Psychotherapy," for which title any neuropsychiatrist, internist, or other specialist could qualify after several years of additional training.

PROBLEMS OF CHILD NEUROPSYCHIATRY

K. Leonhard published a number of works in this field also.[6] It is his conclusion in an important monograph that diagnostics in the field of abnormal child behavior is still quite imprecise. The reason may be sought in the lack of knowledge of children's personalities, their differentiation, and their ways of reacting. To fill this gap, he conducted studies to determine how far a child's neurosis may be considered a true product of milieu injury and how much it reflects deviation of the child's personality. Concerning child neurosis due to educational injuries, he describes in their neurotogenic effects the main forms: brutality in upbringing, narrowing of the overall vital space, alternating over-strict and over-permissive upbringing, over-protection, and the lack of upbringing. Child neuroses due to personality traits is also described in sixteen specific forms of child neuroses due to personality traits in detail and he mentions another two (sensohypochondriacal and autistic traits) which are of no particular importance for child neuroses. Starting from child personality and following up with an investigation of the external damaging factors, an understanding of children's abnormal attitudes may be gained; these he divides into thirteen groups (pathologic opposition, pathologic lack of inhibitions, pathologic jealousy, pathologic fear, etc.). Here again the particular characteristic of Leonhard's work becomes apparent: his attempt at obtaining numerous maximally delimited subforms. He explains his orientation by asserting that specific therapy is possible only if all specific forms are considered with maximal differentiation.

G. Göllnitz, C. Wieck and L. Eichler are among the leading specialists of child neuropsychiatry in the GDR. Göllnitz, who heads the University Clinic in Rostock, has made it an important center for study and practice in this field. He specifically examined the problem of early brain damage. He also contributed important works on functional disturbances in childhood, rehabilitative instruction, and the therapy of children with brain damage.

C. Wieck devoted fifteen years of continuous work to raise the pediatric department of the Nerve Clinic of Leipzig University to its acknowledged high level. In his own work he has attempted to define schizophrenia in childhood as a rare but clearly differentiable affection by applying precise differential diagnostics to distinguish it from schizophrenia-like syndromes and child autism.[26] He reports extensively on his considerable clinical experience, including long-term catamneses of numerous pediatric patients. These yield a rather unfavorable prognosis despite intensive repeated therapy with insulin, chemotherapy, and psychotherapeutic measures consisting mainly in directed play therapy and group and milieu therapy.

Mrs. L. Eichler, who heads the mental hospital at Görden, has made important contributions to the therapy and rehabilitation of retarded children and adolescents. By applying conditioned-reflex methods, she has been able to teach manual dexterity to many children and juveniles who had earlier been considered ineducable, and she could thus regulate their behavior and often enable them to engage in work activities.

Organizational provisions have been made in the GDR to assure early diagnostic records of ineducable retarded children and to make these children benefit in time from special instruction. A network of special schools has been created in all districts of the Republic; these have recently been provided with facilities for varied technical instruction. E. Bartsch has shown in her doctoral thesis, "The Importance of the Production Training for Development and Progress in Retarded School Children," that simultaneous judicious use of mental and motor functions, as required for combining the usual instruction with that for artisan and industrial activities, causes no over-exertion in retarded juveniles; rather, a distinct increase in performance is seen. Their self-confidence is raised and mental balance is obtained. The important results of Dr. E. Bartsch's work are apt to show new ways for achieving optimal educational and therapeutic effects in mildly retarded children and juveniles.

BORDERLINE PROBLEMS

In several of his works Müller-Hegemann attempted to discuss the damaging effects exterted on psychiatry by the fascist dictatorship. These papers[18, 12] were occasioned by doubts concerning the interpretation of a law, dated September 29, 1950, providing for the interruption of pregnancy because of hereditary disease. He explained in them that it would be wrong to overlook a number of diseases which are strongly conditioned by hereditary factors and could, therefore, justify interruption of pregnancy. This would apply only to the individual case where severe hereditary disease could be expected with a high degree of probability. He stressed the basic difference between this law and eugenics, which developed from the erroneous application of Darwin's teachings to human conditions and turned into race biology, i.e., the idea of breeding a presumably superior human race. The latter became the "scientific" weapon for the mass killing of human beings by the German fascist rulers. He mentioned A. Hoche's publication (in collaboration with K. Binding), "The Release of Worthless Human Life for Annihilation" and the lack of public critical reaction by Germany's medical profession after World War I.

Early and sharp rejection of inhuman theories in medicine is required, for only after any kind of eugenics or race biology has been clearly defined and rejected can we proceed with the investigation of hereditary disease and its practical conclusions without being haunted by the past. That such discussions are still timely may be seen from the fact that W. Catel, Ordinary for pediatrics at Kiel after the end of World War II, published in 1962 a paper[2] where he tried to defend ending the life of infant idiots. In this case, the reaction in both Germanies of the medical profession, directed toward refuting infractions against the basic rules of medical ethics, was much more pronounced than it had been after the publication of the book by Hoche and Binding.

Basic problems of philosophy and psychology were raised in the course of a discussion in the periodical "Psychiatrie, Neurologie and Medizinische Psychologie." This was started by C. Weinschenk (Marburg, West Germany) with publication of the paper "The Site of Consciousness,"[25] in which he claimed that consciousness as an ideational re-creation is a function of the brain; he located it in the brain trunk, specifically in the reticular substance, according to results obtained in Magoun's studies. Dagobert Muller of Berlin took the opposite view.[11] He argued that the prerequisites for consciousness, i.e., the sharpness of sensory functions as according to Weinschenk's concept of vigilance, had been mistaken for consciousness, and that Weinschenk's concept would reduce consciousness to physiological or biological data. Human consciousness is not a biologic he argued and is but a social product, thus a subjective reflection of objective reality.

Müller-Hegemann also took part in this discussion.[15] He referred the argument to clinical experience. He described a young patient who had undergone thorough examination; the patient was unable to speak but possessed a limited ability for ordered, correlated ideation.[9] He revealed no consciousness as a social product, but his integrated, correlated mental functions bearing on the solution of important vital tasks far exceeded vigilance. Empirically based arguments were brought forth against both Weinschenk's and Müller's concepts, and the idea of levels of consciousness was advanced: on the lowest level, consciousness may be said to correspond to vigilance as seen in the infant. Here most probably its localization in the brain trunk may be assumed. As the child develops into an adult who is fully responsible and able to function in modern society, consciousness will also develop until it becomes the main regulatory factor of human behavior. These highly complex mental functions would have to be linked primarily to the cerebral hemispheres, and sharp localization would seem impossible. Thus, consciousness is both a biologically and (on the higher levels) socially determined phenomenon.

There exists no survey on medical psychology in the GDR. We would, however, mention a short monograph by Leonhard entitled "Biological Psychology,"[5] because he discusses several psychological fundamentals in this work. He defines psychology as "the conscious faculty or at least conscious attempt to understand human behavior in life and show the ways which lead to this behavior." In his opinion, nothing basic has changed in experimental psychology since Dilthey's critical evaluation; all psychology based mainly on experiments is extraneous to life. Psychology, including experimental psychology, is essentially rooted in the method of self-observation. He also deals with the problem "consciousness and the subconscious," with human instincts and drives for which he lists many subforms, with sensations and emotions, volition, ideational associations, and the powers of intelligence.

Forensic psychiatry is a socially important borderline field, and a large number of papers have been published in the professional press. H. Szewczyk* deserves praise for organizing symposia with international participation in 1963 and 1964, rallying a large number of psychiatrists, forensic physicians, jurists, psychologists, and other scientists. The collection,[24] edited by H. Szewczyk, gives a survey on the 1963 symposium. From details reported in this publication it may be seen that a new penal law is being prepared in the GDR; the basically important Paragraph 51 of the penal code concerning the sanity of the defendant is going to be

---

* Director of the Department of Judicial Psychiatry of the Nerve Clinic at the Charité, Berlin.

changed. The discussions dealt with the advisability of retaining the two subdivisions of the paragraph, Section 1 (not responsible because of severe psychiatric affections) and Section 2 (limited responsibility because of mild psychiatric affections) and with the desirability of new formulations. Problems of penal law for juveniles and of civil law (particularly guardianship procedures) were repeatedly discussed. The 1964 symposium was valuable in that a number of foreign psychiatrists and jurists reported on conditions in their countries. Collaboration between jurists and judicial psychiatrists was improved as a result of these meetings; this may be seen from the fact that psychiatrists are now more frequently called in as consultants in court trials. In such cases the judiciary demands that the psychiatrist elucidate as far as possible the evolution of the defendant's personality in contribution to an understanding of his misdeeds and that he also advise on possible therapeutic measures.

The important borderline fields of "mental hygiene" and "social psychiatry" were the subjects of two meetings at Leipzig. The first topic was debated by the Regional Society for Psychiatry and Neurology[22] in 1960. Papers were presented on "History and Present State of Endeavors Toward Mental Hygiene," "Noise in the City and Its Importance for the Central Nervous System," "The Role of Interpersonal Relations for the Mental Health of the Child," "Mental Hygiene and School Education," "Mental Hygiene in the Adolescent," "Mental Hygiene During Pregnancy and Confinement," "Mental Hygiene in the Psychiatric Hospital," and "Mental Hygiene and Old Age." Increasing attention was given to the problem of "mental health" in the GDR as a result of this meeting.

The second meeting, organized by the Society for Medical Psychotherapy, which took place in 1961, was reported in a paper[17] by D. Müller-Hegemann. In reference to the earlier mentioned study about persons with hearing difficulties, it was reported that examination of 380 individuals from a representative selection of such cases revealed ten percent suffering from psychoses or other affections (depressions and paranoid manifestations); depressive neuroses lacking the character of disease were excluded. Forty percent had no relevant psychiatric manifestations. It was thus concluded that the percentage of mental disease is distinctly higher in the partly deaf than in the average population and also that successful rehabilitation of the deaf by means of modern hearing aids and particularly by fitting these persons into a suitable social environment can easily be accomplished.

The "Serial Studies of Individuals Persecuted by the Nazi Regime" on 100 carefully examined individuals who had spent a long time in solitary confinement showed that the majority suffered from its sequelae (nervous, cardiovascular, and other disturbances), but that they were able to tolerate the enormous strain of solitary confinement by continuously doing gymnastics and mnemonics and by communicating with other prisoners (rapping signals). These observations were not generalized, since they concerned an unusual selection of former prisoners. It was also found that even the most determined will to resist discovers its limits if the solitary prisoner is put in chains for a long time, i.e., deprived of motor function. The fate of such a prisoner was described; he had been perfectly healthy until his fortieth year but acquired incurable schizophrenia after such imprisonment.

W. Barthel reported on "Neuropsychiatric Studies in Leipzig Telephone Operators." Thirty percent suffered from neurasthenia, but the anamneses showed no significant excess in illness over other groups of workers.

W. Funke conducted "Serial Studies on the Frequency of Common Complaints"; seventy-eight percent of the 117 individuals examined had no organic disease and felt well on the day they were examined. Upon closer questioning, seventy-one percent of these complained of functional disorders. When the question was phrased suggestively, this percentage increased to ninety-three percent. Complaints referred mainly to vegetative functions, static sensations, cardiovascular functions, and rheumatic phenomena, although no pathological disorders were seen in the great majority. This illustrates the importance of the phrasing of questions and the danger that neuroses and other disturbances may be postulated as mass phenomena.

OUTLOOK

Neurology and psychiatry are still being treated as just one discipline in the GDR; except for Rostock University, there exists only a single chair at each of the universities providing for uniform training in the specialty. Thus, uniformly trained specialists are available for central and peripheral organizations. However, as in West Germany, more and more voices are heard pleading for a division into two or even three disciplines: neurology, psychiatry, and pediatric neuropsychiatry. The main reasons given are the constantly increasing amount of scientific material and certain differences of method in the direction of neurological and psychiatric investigation and work. The board of directors of the Society for Psychiatry and Neurology has failed to support this opinion; while admitting that further specialization is urgently required, it pointed to the dangers of over-specialization without simultaneous coordination of such specialities and of losing sight of the basic links. In severe disease, the brain, the most important organ for both neurology and psychiatry, is the source of both somatic and psychic manifestations; frequently occurring affections (cerebral vascular disease, epilepsy, involutional brain processes) as well as neuroses permit no primary division into neurological and psychiatric sectors. It has also been said that the psychiatrist who has had no thorough neurological training and subsequent neurological practice may easily succumb to the danger of psychologism, just as the highly specialized neurologist may be unaware of the many psychopathological aspects of brain disease.

There is agreement that the neuropsychiatrist, following a thorough, well-rounded training, should find his special area of studies, which would be much more limited than the field of psychiatry or neurology. These questions are still under debate, and future developments cannot be anticipated.

Both psychiatrists and neurologists in the GDR agree on the need for a larger role of their specialty within the field of general medicine. The concept of the human being as a whole, the manifold psychological and also philosophical problems proper to this discipline, should be of great importance to every modern physician in his everyday work, whatever organs it may involve, whether he is a surgeon or an anatomist. Other important fields are those of rehabilitation, whose psychological aspects require just as much attention as the physical, and the promotion of "mental health" at a time of technical and social revolution. This requires the help of every physician. Only on this basis will it be possible to engage the public interest for optimally complete health protection.

References

1. E. BARTHEL, D. MULLER-HEGEMANN, AND B. SCHWARTZ: Series of Investigations of Hard-of-Hearing Individuals within the Scope of the City of Leipzig, *Psychiatry*, (10) (1962).
2. W. CATEL: "Marginal Life Situation, Contribution to the Problem of Limited Euthanasia," Nuremberg, 1962.
3. G. GOLLNITZ: "The Importance of Early Brain Damage for Child Psychiatry," Leipzig, 1954.
4. H. KLEINSORGE AND G. KLUMBIES: "Psychotherapy in Clinic and Practice," Munich and Berlin, 1959.
5. K. LEONHARD: "Biological Psychology," Leipzig, 1961.
6. K. LEONHARD: "Child Neurosis and Child Personality," Berlin, 1963.
7. K. LEONHARD: "Individual Therapy and Prophylaxis of Hysterical, Anankastic, and Sensohypochondriacal Neuroses," Jena, 1959.
8. K. LEONHARD AND V. TROSTORFF: "Prognostic Diagnoses of Endogenetic Psychoses," Jena, 1964.
9. G. MEIER AND D. MÜLLER-HEGEMANN: Linguistic and Neuropsychiatric Studies in a Lone Type, Incapable of Speech, *Psychiatrie, Neurologie und Med. Psychologie*, (6):203 (1961).
10. A. METTE: "Sigmund Freud," Berlin, 1956.
11. D. MÜLLER-HEGEMANN: Remarks on "The Site of Consciousness," *Psychiatrie, Neurologie und Med. Psychologie*, (12):52 (1960).
12. D. MÜLLER-HEGEMANN: The Effect of Eugenics on German Medicine, *Das Deutsche Gesundheitswesen [German Public Health]*, 14:429 (1959).
13. D. MÜLLER-HEGEMANN: Methodical Approaches in Psychotherapy, *Amer. J. of Psychotherapy*, 17:554 (1963).
14. D. MÜLLER-HEGEMANN: "Neurology and Psychiatry," Berlin, 1966.
15. D. MÜLLER-HEGEMANN: The Problem of Human Consciousness, *Psychiatrie, Neurologie und Med. Psychologie*, (13):212 (1961).
16. D. MÜLLER-HEGEMANN: "Psychotherapie," Berlin, 1961.
17. D. MÜLLER-HEGEMANN: Some Acute Problems of Social Psychiatry, *Int. J. Soc. Psych.*, 9(3):216 (1963). [Report of the Society for Medical Psychotherapy meeting of October 2–3, 1961.]
18. D. MÜLLER-HEGEMANN: Theoretical Bases of the Indication for Interruption of Pregnancy because of Hereditary Disease, *Das Deutsche Gesundheitswesen*, 10:241 (1955).
19. D. MÜLLER-HEGEMANN, ed.: "Present Problems of Hypnosis," Leipzig, 1964. [Contains a report of the 1962 meeting of the Society for Medical Psychotherapy.]
20. "Problems of Neurosis in Clinic and Experiment," Volk und Gesundheit, Berlin, 1959. [Collection of readings including contributions by the major neuropsychiatrists and other medical specialists practicing in the GDR.]
21. Report of the 1963 Congress for Psychiatry, Dresden, *Psychiatrie, Neurologie und Med. Psychologie*, (3), 1965.

22. Report of the Regional Society of Psychiatry and Neurology, Leipzig, June 9–10, 1960, *Psychiatrie, Neurologie und Med. Psychologie,* (13):28 (1961).

23. H. SIMON: Active Treatment of Patients in the Sanitarium, *Allg. Z. Psychiatrie [General Journal of Psychiatry]*, 87 and 90.

24. H. SZEWCZYK, ed.: "Judicial Psychiatry under the New Judiciary System," Jena, 1964.

25. C. WEINSCHENK: The Site of Consciousness, *Psychiatrie, Neurologie und Med. Psychologie,* (12):43 (1960).

26. C. WIECK: "Schizophrenia in Childhood," Leipzig, 1965.

CHAPTER FOUR

The History of Hungarian Psychiatry: An Outline

BY
DR. GYULA NYIRÖ

THE DEVELOPMENT OF HUNGARIAN psychiatry is divided into a pre-scientific and a scientific period. The former was characterized by various magical and mystical ideas about mental disease. From the year 1015 we have documentary evidence that in the Benedictine monastery at Pécs-várad, prayers, laying-on of hands, and exorcism were used as treatments for the insane. Later documents contain more and more allusions to the insane; in addition to the often inhuman methods used to deal with them, there is increasing evidence of a more sober, humanistic attitude and a genuine desire to help them. In the use of herbs for the cure of various mental disorders there is a definite attempt at scientific, causal treatment. Such an approach is presented, for example, in the eighteenth-century work of Veszprémi. A major turning point was the gradual introduction of mental hospitals into the country. Earlier, mental patients were confined to poorhouses, prisons, and various asylums; in the mental hospitals there was, for the first time, the possibility of their treatment in accordance with the principles of scientific medicine. Due to the ideas of Pinel it became increasingly clear in Hungarian medical circles that mental patients, instead of having to be restrained by various punishments derived from philosophical speculation, should be treated by doctors.

Although Pest County requested the establishment of a separate mental ward within the county hospital as early as 1801 and later applied for a separate mental institution, the first so-called "insane asylum" did not come into being until 1840. Its establishment was due to the private initiative of József Pólya. But after functioning for a short time under strict limitations, the institution was closed down. During the first half of the nineteenth century mental patients were treated in the public hospitals. Some attempts at a diagnostic approach were made at the Satoraljaujhely hospital: in classifying psychotics the doctors endeavored to separate mental disorders that could be traced to physical causes from those that were of a psychological origin.

MODERN HUNGARIAN PSYCHIATRY TO 1945

The beginnings of scientific psychiatry in Hungary can be fixed in the year 1850. It was in that year that Ferenc Schwartzer opened his private mental hospital. In 1858 Schwartzer published a textbook on psychiatry, which approached mental disorders from an anatomical and neurological point of view.

In the second half of the nineteenth century the country saw the rapid building of several large mental hospitals. In 1863 one was opened in Nagyszeben, followed by one in Budapest and one in Nagykálló. Ernö Emil Moravcsik and Károly Lechner, both pupils of Schwartzer, were the first to make Hungarian psychiatry internationally known. Moravcsik gained recognition mainly by his research on hallucinations. In his experiments he produced hallucinations by various stimuli (tuning fork, pinpricks, colored objects) and concluded that the delusions thus produced were not necessarily in the area of the stimulated sense organ. He also observed that the delusion would always be a part of the pathological picture. He believed that the formation of hallucinations involves, beside the important peripheral elements, a change in the workings of the entire cortex. Hallucinations reach their full development, he suggested, where there is a dissociation of consciousness. He also tried to establish quantitative relationships between the stimulus, on the one hand, and the strength and progress of the delusion, on the other. His studies extended to hysteria, paranoia, and paralysis progressiva, and he also gave a description of the hyperpyrexia and delirious disturbances associated with rabies. In criminal psychiatry he was mainly interested in paranoic states resulting from imprisonment and also in alcoholism. Moravcsik also gave a description of certain grotesque movements produced by epileptic patients in their state of euphoria and hyperthymia. He gave them the name of *euthymopraxia.* As a university professor he taught neurology and psychiatry in Budapest for many years. His textbook went through several editions and was the accepted guide for medical students and specialists in the country.

Károly Lechner intended to put psychiatry on an independent footing. Like Wernicke, he had wished to establish an organic basis for psychiatry in certain pathological processes. In his rigorous application of the results obtained from the observation of reflexes, he was among the first on the international scene to connect psychic events to physiological processes. According to Lechner, psychic changes are physiological changes and, like all other physiological developments, are derived from the physical modifications of cells. He called the cells "miniature energy centers" and compared the intercellular changes to the explosion of gunpowder. Just as energy is liberated in gunpowder by the spark, so certain stimuli liberate energy in the cell. The manifestations of this energy are heat, chemical changes, electricity, movement, etc.

The difference between the two kinds of energy releases is that the process within the cells has an additional energy component that is never present in the transformations of inorganic matter. This component is *feeling.* Feeling is an irreducible, basic phenomenon. According to Lechner's hypothesis, every living organism represents a particular energy system. As a result of inner or outer stimuli, the homeostasis of the system is disturbed, and the disturbance is registered as *excitement.* Excitement is the general property of living matter. Generally speaking, wherever there is life, there is excitability. Wherever there is a reaction, wherever there is adaptation, that is to say a kind of selection between the necessary stimuli on the one hand and a variety of reactions on the other, there is excitation in response to the stimuli. Adaptation presupposes feeling, because a selective response is only possible if the stimuli are conveyed through feeling. The stimulus and the response are linked by the reflex.

Lechner distinguishes four kinds of reflexes. The simplest are the completely unconscious cellular reflexes. Complex tasks such as swallowing may be accomplished by half-conscious cellular chain reactions. From the linkage of organ chain reactions conscious organ-bound reflexes are formed, such as attention, remembering, and conscious action. The fourth kind of reflex is mechanical reflex action (reading, writing, walking, speech).

According to Lechner's hypothesis, the various kinds of these four reflex types occur massively in man. By their intricate interaction they form reflex complexes that manifest themselves in mental activity and emotion. Under the influence of disease the reflexes may diminish *in toto*, or else they may increase. In the event of greater incorporation of stimuli, their reaction may diminish, or the opposite may occur. These four types of diseased reflexes can form both by assimilation and by dissimilation. Lechner's reflex theory, which he formed independently of Bechterev and also before Pavlov, was very suitable for organizing and interpreting the accumulating results of psychiatric data collection available in his time. His theory about sleep and dreams was adopted by Bing.

As against Lechner's characteristically independent views, the various psychiatric approaches prevalent in Europe at the time have also had their direct influence in Hungary. Gyula Donáth recommended fever therapy for paralysis progressiva. Wagner von Jauregg of Vienna later developed his own method of fever therapy. Donáth was also active in exploring the anatomy of the frontal lobe and he was known for his research in pharmacology and ophthalmology. He was editor of the international periodical *Epilepsia* and a leader in the campaign against alcoholism. The name of Jakab Salgó is remembered for his textbook on psychopathology published in 1882. Jenó Konrád was director of the Lipotmezo mental hospital in Budapest; he worked mainly in the areas of paralysis progressiva and the mental disorders of children. Artur Sarbó was an investigator of the pathology of syphilis, epilepsy, and speech disorders.

During the first decades of the twentieth century three main trends can be identified in Hungarian psychiatry. The strongest of these was cerebral pathology, but the experimental psychiatry pursued by the Institute of Child Psychology and the depth-psychological approach also had their adherents. The development of research in cerebral pathology was mainly the work of Károly Schaffer. While professor at Budapest University, Schaffer established a laboratory for research in cerebral pathology. He issued regular publications about his own as well as about his assistants' research. The anatomical foundations of idiotia amaurotica familiaris were clarified by him, for which reason this disorder if often called the Tay-Sachs-Schaffer disease. In his textbook on neurology and psychopathology he juxtaposed neurological and psychological disorders, because he believed that in the ultimate analysis one cannot sharply separate the organic diseases of the nervous system from psychic disorders. Miskolczy and Horányi worked on histological correlations of schizophrenia at Schaffer Institute.

They postulated an abiotrophic process as the basic phenomenon. Although the results of their research were discarded later, their explorations provided starting points for many subsequent research projects.

Professor Kálmán Sántha, a pioneer of Hungarian neurosurgery, was also Schaffer's pupil. His research in psychiatry centered primarily on problems of the psychoorganic syndrome and on the border areas of neuropsychiatry, but his early death prevented him from working out a synthesis of his lifetime research. Laszlo Benedek was also essentially a follower of the school of cerebral pathology. His lasting work lies mainly in the area of organic brain syndrome. He is internationally known for his research on the Korszakov syndrome. He devoted much attention to the clinical manifestations and the psychopathology of the diencephalon. Within this area he was specially interested in the problem of sleep and in the excitation of the brainstem. His observations on the occipital and parietal lobes are also of permanent value. He published some work in the area of combat neuroses, and as a lecturer he was internationally known. József Szabó devoted himself to investigating the identification fallacies of memory and collaborated on a textbook of psychopathology with the author of this report.

The work of Laszlo Meduna should also be mentioned here. Basing his treatment on studies by Nyirö and Jablonszky, Meduna made use of the known antagonism between schizophrenia and epilepsy. First he used injections of camphor and later of cardiazol to produce convulsions in the patients. Although his treatment was later superseded by the electric-shock treatment, his discovery was epoch-making in the history of psychiatry. His later work is significant mainly for the description he gave of oneirophrenia as an independent form of disease.

The investigations of István Környey, professor at the University of Pécs, centered around the clinical pathology of the Korszakov syndrome. These studies likewise belong to the organic school. His internationally known investigations on vasal damages due to lack of oxygen have a significance in psychopathology as well. One of the most outstanding representatives of the Schaffer school is Dezsö Miskolczy, who held professorial chairs at Szeged, Kolozsvár, and Marosvásárhely and is now professor at the Postdoctoral Studies Institute in Budapest. He became internationally known through his histological research on schizophrenia, his studies of presenile and senile changes, and his many publications. During the fifties he published a textbook. While professor at Kolozsvár, he established there a department of neurosurgery.

Pál Büchler made some significant contributions in his investigations of connections between the functional disorders of the liver and mental disease as well as between hormone disorders and psychopathological symptoms. Endre Kluge succeeded in circumscribing the pathography of paranoia imitata. He gave this name to the manic disorders manifested by paranoid persons. He described the phenomenon of the voluntary and gradual generation of a state of rage, which usually occurs in psychopaths, although it may be observed in normal individuals as well.

Among the psychiatrists of organic orientation Professor Lajor Angyal occupies a special position. He followed Kleist regarding the various kinds of schizophrenia as organic diseases of the brain and used subtle, symptomatic analysis to describe well-delineated components of the disease. Angyal gave a detailed description of insulin shock, distinguishing six phases and four types. Using these observations and histological research, he attempted on the one hand to localize symptoms of schizophrenia and on the other to determine the degree of regression in the workings of the central nervous system.

Professor Pál Ranschburg established the Institute of Child Psychology, which produced some excellent research in experimental psychology. Ranschburg made himself known by describing the phenomenon of homogenous inhibition. He did extensive research on memory, attributing an important role to homogenous concept inhibition in the mechanisms of memory. He also modified Ziehen's word-pair test. He followed Moravcsik in stimulating hallucinations and investigated extensively the laws of concept building. Among his works dealing with child psychology, his studies on legasthenia, or writing and reading defects, and on counting are outstanding. Ranschburg established a school of followers in Hungary.

Among the various trends of depth psychology, Freudian psychoanalysis gained the most adherents in Hungary. Sándor Ferenczy was one of the most prominent representatives of orthodox psychoanalysis. He was known for his description of the phenomenon of introjection and its analytical elaboration. Istvan Hollós was also oriented toward psychoanalysis, but in addition to his work as a psychoanalyst he also investigated the problems of paranoia and epilepsy. With his *Farewell to the Yellow House,* a novel, he introduced Hungarian psychiatry into the world of *belles lettres.* In his medical practice he was characterized by a most scrupulously humanistic attitude. Imre Hermann was mainly preoccupied with the primary and secondary processes of thinking. The ideas of C. G. Jung were represented in Hungary by Jolán Jacobi. Among the various depth-psychological approaches, Lipót Szondi and his pupils formed an independent school. Szondi, whose later work was done in Zurich, developed a singular theory of instincts. He believed that the various kinds of instincts may be determined by analysing photographs of the mentally ill, of psychopaths, and of neurotics, which he collected for this purpose. He called his method *fate analysis*. Both his followers and his critics are numerous. From the beginning, the psychoanalytical school was sharply criticized in Hungary; its excesses were opposed by Lechner, Ranschburg, and Benedek.

A separate place is reserved within the history of Hungarian psychiatry for the attempts to improve the accommodation, care, and rehabilitation of the mentally ill. Most of the mental institutions built after the middle of the nineteenth century did not fulfill the hopes of humanists. As institutions all over the world, initially they had the character of prisons and the patients were often subjected to force (strait jackets, etc.). The "no-restraint principle," first advocated by Connolly, has found adherents in Hungary. Such was Gyula Niedermann (1840–1910), who followed this principle in governmental institutions and led the fight for more humane methods of treatment. Though Niedermann's work did bring some results, the real change was brought about by Gusztáv Oláh. Oláh abolished the defamatory title of "madhouse" and established parks, playing fields, lounges, and workshops for the patients. He wrote separate studies on how to build mental hospitals and on the problems of care for the patients. In 1900, he gave a lecture in Paris, where he outlined a program for the Movement for Mental Hygiene initiated by Toulouse. In 1924, he organized the Hungarian League for the Protection of the Mentally Ill. The basic tenets of the League were that instead of putting the mentally ill under guard, efforts should be made to prevent their becoming ill; in case of illness, efforts should be made to cure them. "It is the cell that makes the cell necessary" in a mental institution was his memorable remark. At the age of seventy, Oláh presented a proposal for settling the legal status of the mentally ill. This deeply humanistic proposal was made into a law in Norway. Apart from his work in these areas, he wrote a book, *Genius and Insanity*, in which he investigated the connections between the two.

A peculiarly Hungarian endeavor was the so-called "hospitalization movement," championed by Gusztáv Oláh, Zoltán A. Rath, and Imre Szecsödy. They contended that treatment of the mentally ill in separate institutions tends to brand them and inhibit their return to society. Therefore they recommended that instead of building self-contained mental institutions, the general hospitals should establish wards for psychotics in the same complex of buildings where other patients are treated.

In the early 1920's Oláh began the campaign for the establishment of an institute for the care of the mentally ill. The work was completed by Rudolf Fabinyi. The institute created is concerned not only with the prevention of mental illness but also with the aftercare of patients. By keeping a complete file on each patient, the hospital has a detailed and realistic picture of the patient's family and social circumstances. The social worker's task includes instruction for as well as rehabilitation work with the cured patient. One of Fabinyi's published writings deals with care for the mentally ill within the family. He also urged bringing mental health statistics up to date and organizing a school for nurses of mental patients. In his institutional practice he believed in the early discharge of mental patients.

Pál Pándy also played an active part in the organization of home care for patients and in the establishment of colonies. He was *privatdozent* at the University of Budapest and internationally famous for the globulin reaction named after him, which he originally believed to be a specific characteristic of syphilis.

HUNGARIAN PSYCHIATRY FROM
WORLD WAR II TO THE PRESENT

During World War II, Hungarian psychiatry suffered seemingly irreparable losses. Such was the death of Professor László Benedek, director of the Psychiatric and Neurological Hospital of the University of Budapest. Also, many of the psychiatric institutes suffered great physical damages from the war. However, reconstruction began almost immediately, the hospitals were restaffed, the patients were traced and institutionalized, and by the end of 1945 the network of psychiatric institutions was beginning to grow. Centers for work therapy were also established.

Due to the enormous changes in the country's social structure as reflected in the scientific world view and in the ideological revolution, emphasis after the war shifted to neurophysiological research and Pavlovian reflex studies. As a result, the split between the psychoorganic and purely psychological research was somewhat diverted from the physiological, biochemical, electrophysiological, and, especially, structural-dynamic fields, which were cultivated by clinicians and researchers who followed the traditions of the great Hungarian schools of psychology (Ranschburg, Lechner, etc.). The demands of social reconstruction gave considerable momentum to psychological research, especially in the fields of labor organization, educational psychology, and rehabilitation. The concrete problems and organizational methods of mental care and mental health administration are reflected in a large part of post-war literature (Angyal, Bálint, Hollós, Csekey, L. Tóth, Juhász, Lehoczky, Stief). Hungarian psychiatry continued to develop along the new organizational principles in the national institute, in the psychiatric wards of various hospitals, and in the mental hospitals of Szeged, Pécs, and Debrecen. The same development took place in the regional mental health centers and in the work-therapy institutions. Between 1945 and 1951, there was no unified school of psychiatry. Groups of researchers and projects were moving in different directions in the various university centers: in Budapest neuropathology was stressed, in Szeged biochemistry, in Debrecen electrophysiology, and in Pécs neurophysiology.

Because of circumstances characteristic of Hungary, research in child psychiatry was mainly carried on in Budapest, primarily in pediatric and psychological directions. Because of this concentration in Budapest, a unified organization of child psychiatric care came into being only very slowly, although excellent workers like Margit Révész and Blanka Loránd were connected with it.

Already before World War II, and after the death of Fabinyi, a committee of four took over the organization of mental health administration in Budapest and in the nation at large. At that time the committee was chaired by Budapest's health commissioner, Csordás. After the war, the so-called "Health Council" was formed, first with seven and then ten permanent members.

From 1951 onwards, Nyirö built a school of followers around himself. He based his psychophysiological theories on the reflexology of the Hungarian Károly Lechner and of I. Pavlov. Nyirö regarded the nervous system as a complex organization of chemodynamics without knowledge of which response formation and extinction cannot be understood. He also recognized the structural laws of evolution and the hierarchy of phylogenetic development in psychic processes.

He believed that in the formation of man's psychic activities, the differentiation between object- and self-consciousness is essential. The physiological formation of psychic activities follows those processes which

Pavlov recognized as the basic principles of the physiological activities of the nervous system: structuralism, determinism, and finally, the principle of analysis and synthesis. According to Nyirö's theory, then, the organization of psychic activities within the framework of reflex processes takes on a threefold structure. This structuring becomes ever more differentiated during the ontogenetic development. The activities connected with cognition, relating, and adaptation become parts of separate mechanisms. Within individual organizations, but also interorganizationally, temporal linkages are established. If these linkages are biologically useful for longer periods of time, they become dynamic stereotypes. These latter are identifiable with the chains of conditioned reflexes already known to us from physiology.

Between the temporal and permanent functional organizations, lower- and higher-level linkages are formed. Among these the linkages which are repeated in identical forms and establish shortened circuits to economize on are called "dynamic stereotypes." During the course of development the lower-level stereotypes become increasingly inhibited by the higher-level stereotypes. However, the lower-level stereotypes, being more archaic, more rigid, and more strictly determined (with a narrower base), contain much fewer nervous processes, circuits, and connections. The higher-level stereotypes are looser and more variable. Our lower-level stereotypes show collective characteristics: they become typical of certain communities, sometimes even of individual families. Thus they can become quite restricted, but, on the other hand, they might characterize a whole people. In speaking of structural development we must note that, through the cognitive organization and development of speech, man has become so enriched that he has surpassed all other living beings. The difference between man and other living beings is one not only of degree but also of kind. With the development of the human brain, corticalization shows a variety which cannot be found in other living species. This difference is found in the sensory and motor centers of speech. That there is a qualitative jump in evolution here is shown in the fact that the activity of speech as a whole does not have subcortical centers.

Physiologically a well-defined state of cortical excitability is consciousness, which depends on exteroceptive stimulation from the outside and also on the central tension of readiness (*Antrieb*) generated by interoceptive activity by the inner organs. The latter is especially dependent on the system of brainstem stimulation and on the state of excitement in the hypothalamus. On the basis of these factors a lower and a higher state of consciousness may be established. On the lower level afferent visceral impulses become conscious, whereas on the higher level the stimuli of the second signaling system reach consciousness.

Nyirö derives his psychopathological interpretations from the regressional, dissociational, and conscious changes in the structural hierarchy. He distinguishes the corresponding reversible or irreversible, episodic, reactive, processive, or phasal personality damages or personality distortions. In his detailed psychopathology he deals with psychoses, psychopathic disorders, neuroses, and oligophrenia, as well as disorders due to exogenous reactions. Within all these groups he validates the dynamic structural view, according to which both endogenous and exogenous genetic factors can produce these changes by tight interaction. In his classification of neuroses he talks of situational-conflict, exhaustive, and purposive neuroses, which fall symptomatically into groups of neurasthenia, psychasthenia, and hysteria. He classifies the persons suffering from psychopathic disorders as "thymopaths," "characteropaths," "telopaths," and "instinct psychopaths."

Nyirö's psychiatric work in the criminal courts gave him much experience and enabled him to approach real situations according to the structural view outlined above, in a dialectical spirit, without dogmatism or scholasticism. His conviction in both theory and practice is that it is extremely important to establish whether the crime was committed by the individual or by the disease. In his opinion primacy should be given not to exact and immediate diagnosis but to the establishment and clarification of the connection between the consciousness of the perpetrator of the criminal act and the act with which he is being charged.

Nyirö's structural view determines his clinical and psychopathological practice as well as his research and teaching. Together with his coworkers, he investigates in depth the problems of repeated electric-shock treatment, social psychiatric measurements (neurosis, deprivation, etc.), functional disorders of the diencephalon, and endocrinology. Other research by the same group is concerned with psychopathology in border areas, psychiatry in the criminal courts, clinical investigations of psychopharmacology, compulsions, connections between exogeny and endogeny and the measurement of the effectiveness of testing methods employed in clinical psychiatry.

After World War II, the teaching of psychiatry was conducted in

Budapest by the Department of Neurology and Psychiatry until 1957, when the department was divided in two. From that day on, fifth-year medical students had to take a semester of psychiatry ending in a final examination. Since September, 1964, this final examination has been transferred to the sixth year and is given after two weeks of clinical practice in a mental hospital. According to the tradition of Hungarian medical teaching, neurology and psychiatry have been taught within the framework of internal medicine. At the provincial universities the two fields have not yet been separated and both subjects are still taught in the same department.

The nationwide training of specialists is done by the Postdoctoral Studies Institute in Budapest. After concluding a period of professional training subsequent to the completion of his university studies, the new doctor may be qualified as a specialist in psychiatry or in neurology or in both fields together. Before he can be admitted to the first examination in his special field, he is required to work and study in the field for four years. Before the second qualifying examination another two years of specialized practice are necessary.

SOME STATISTICAL DATA

In the following we wish to present a few significant data from representative Hungarian mental health statistics.

During the last few decades an increasing number of persons have suffered from mental and nervous disorders, especially in highly industrialized countries. In Hungary, too, there is a large increase of patients with mental and nervous disorders, both in the hospital wards and in the clinics. Within the last five years alone, the number of patients discharged from mental and neurological institutions and wards has risen by 23 percent. The frequency of mental and nervous disorders is, on the average, 352 per 100,000 persons; this is calculated by the number of patients admitted to institutions or clinics. Men figure among the patients 6.3 percent more frequently than women. More than one-third of the treated persons are suffering from insanity, 29 percent from neuroses, and nearly one-third have been treated for various character, behavior, and intelligence disorders. Although insanity and neurosis are more frequent among women, the total of character, behavior, and intelligence disorders is two and one-half times higher among men. The most frequent form of insanity is schizophrenia, although senile and cerebral sclerosis and post-menopausal and manic-depressive psychoses are also common. All these together account for about 80 percent of the insanity in Hungary.

Eighty percent of the patients are between the ages of twenty and fifty-nine. Only fourteen percent are sixty years old or older. The high proportion of women patients falling between thirty and forty-nine years of age can be attributed to physiological causes (pregnancy, birth, beginning of the menopause, and also to some other objectively ascertainable circumstances).

Sixty-nine percent of mental patients in institutions were breadwinners, and from 100,000 persons in the population almost twice as many breadwinners as non-earning dependents are treated. Among the male breadwinners, eighty-seven percent were active workers, among the females eighty-two percent. The others received various pensions or annuities.

The number of high school graduates, university graduates, and holders of postgraduate degrees is much higher among the mentally ill than their proportion among the total population would suggest. Among 10,000 white-collar workers, the proportion of mentally ill is one and one-half times greater than that among the same number of blue-collar workers. Within this total, women patients are forty percent more numerous than men. These higher proportions show that more complex, more responsible intellectual work as well as administrative type positions controlling larger mechanisms are significant etiological factors in the development of mental and nervous disorders and particularly of neuroses.

Almost eighty percent of the illnesses were produced by exogenous causes, which divide about equally between biological and psychical factors. Endogenous factors cause about one-third more disorders in women than in men. Within the group whose illness is due to exogenous causes, men's illnesses are more often biological (because of various psychical defects), whereas women's illnesses are due more to psychical causes.

On the average, about thirty-six percent of the patients show a type of mental disorder—or a tendency thereof—which can be traced among blood relations. Of all these cases, forty percent show the disease or related disease forms in one or both parents. In the other sixty percent, mental disease occurred mostly in clusters among the parents, grandparents, and other blood relations in various combinations.

Almost sixteen percent of mental and nervous patients admitted to institutions have a record of one or more attempts at suicide. More than half of these were being treated, at the time of the attempt, for mental illness or neurosis.

PSYCHOPHARMACOLOGICAL RESEARCH

Psychopharmacology is a very young field that has been practiced in Hungary for hardly more than a decade. Major and minor tranquilizers, thymoleptics, and psychoenergetics have gained quick adoption in Hungary after brief trial periods abroad. The Hungarian drug industry has manufactured the equivalents of most drugs which were formerly imported from abroad. Moreover, certain preparations, such as Frenolon (of the perphenazin group), furnished valuable new compounds for therapy. Among the Hungarian pharmacological products of the last few years we might mention the discovery of the new psychoenergizer phenylisopropylamin-HCL, which was synthesized by Knoll and his coworkers in 1964. The clinical testing of this drug is now in progress.

By testing the new drugs on animals and patients, the Hungarian researchers contributed to the clarification of effective mechanisms and therapeutic value. The results generally tended to confirm the opinions presented in the literature of many countries. Among the many who have engaged in this kind of research and testing, we must select for special mention Lajos Angyal, Tibor Lehoczky, and Béla Horányi, who contributed mainly to the clarification of the effect mechanism of chloropromazine and imipramine. Their studies are often referred to in the international literature. The therapeutic effects of elysion upon depressive patients were described by Gyula Nyirö and Mrs. Jenö Irányi. Ferenc Fornádi experimented with lucidril and Albert Szobor with haloperidol. A broadly based comparative statistical evaluation of the various treatments in the therapy of depressions is being carried out by Ervin Varga. He collaborates on this project with an international team of researchers within the framework of the World Health Organization.

Hallucinogens also have been tested in Hungary. There have been experiments with lysergic acid diethylamid, mescalin, and psylobicin and their derivatives. Zoltán Böszörményi and his coworkers were the first to give an account of the experiments on the model psychosis produced by diethyltryptamine, a hallucinogen prepared by Hungarian scientists.

Among biochemical research with psychiatric implications, the work of Istvan Huszak and his associates is of importance. They experimented with indolcompounds from schizophrenic patients. They established that in a twenty-four-hour follow up of the daily evacuation, schizophrenics showed a much larger daily fluctuation in the evacuation of 5-hydroxyindolacetic acid than did the control group. Chromatographic analyses of indolcompounds showed a significant pink spot (with Erlich reagent) only with schizophrenics. About fifty percent of schizophrenics also showed a brown oily spot in the chromatogram. Further analyses are continuing in this direction at the Szeged Neurological and Psychiatric Hospital.

PSYCHIATRIC ASPECTS OF PHYSIOLOGICAL RESEARCH

Hungarian psychiatry from the beginning, was closely linked to physiological research and to the materialistic view. From the early 1950s onward, Pavlov's doctrines had a fertilizing effect on Hungarian psychiatric research. Gyula Nyirö, in the development of his structural dynamic theory, has made use of the results of Pavlov's work. Among the studies dealing with methodology of conditioned reflexes, the work of Nyirö and Ilona Huszár on compulsive neuroses and the investigations of Ervin Varga on psychasthenia and on the pathogenesis of schizophrenia are of significance. As we cannot here enter into the discussion of neurophysiological research during the past few years, we refer the reader to the monographs of Lissák and Endröczy. The emphasis of research in our institution has for the last few years been on diencephalon. Of the psychiatric aspects of uremia Ferenc Fornádi and László Szegedy gave an account. The neuropsychiatric effects of the artificial kidney treatment are being examined by Szegedy.

SOCIAL-PSYCHIATRIC RESEARCH

Only during the last few years have social-psychiatric investigations come into worldwide prominence. As a result, this type of research is very new in Hungary. Reference should be made first of all to the investigations of Pál Juhász and his associates. They have examined the conditions of mental hygiene in villages and observed the neuroses of agricultural workers. Nyirö and Ervin Varga used mathematical-statistical methods to examine the neurotic patients of the Budapest Psychiatric Hospital from the social-psychiatric point of view. Nyirö and his coworkers made analytical studies on the connections between the various forms of psychoses and neuroses among people living in different cultural and climatic environments on the one hand, and between the different social, cultural, and climatic factors on the other.

References

1. L. CSEKEY: "The Progress of Psychiatric Care in the Last Fifty Years, with Special Reference to the Data of Our Hospital," 1950.
2. T. DÁN AND GY. BALÁZS: "The Development of Mental Care in Hungary."
3. I. HARDI: "The Developmental History of Psychotherapy."
4. I. KULCSÁR: "Periods of Mental Hygiene."
5. D. TANKA: "The Last Ten Years in Neurology and Psychiatry," 1957.
6. I. ZSAKÓ: "The History of the Origins of the Former National Lunatic Asylum."
7. M. ZSIGMOND: "The Hospital of Angyalföld."

CHAPTER FIVE

The Development of Psychiatry in Yugoslavia

BY
DR. VLADIMIR JAKOVLJEVIC

THE FRAMEWORK OF THE CULTURAL ENVIRONMENT

YUGOSLAVIA OCCUPIES AN AREA OF 255,804 SQUARE KILOMETERS and extends from the Balkan peninsula to mid-Europe. Geographically it comprises the Adriatic coastline in the west, the Panonic lowland region in the northeast, and the extensive mountain belt in between.

The distribution of the 19,525,000 inhabitants in 1965 ranges from a density of thirty to eighty inhabitants per square kilometer. Density is greatest in towns and industrial centers, less in the lowland and coastline regions, and the least in the mountain regions. There are more women than men, although the ratio of women to men is becoming more and more equal. In 1961 it was 1,064 to 1,000. The age structure of the population is distinguished by a high percentage of children under 15 years of age and a rather low percentage of population above 45 years of age, although the number of older persons is gradually increasing. In 1961, 35 percent of the population was under 15 years of age, 44 percent between 15 and 44, and only 25 percent older than 45. This age structure is the result of high birth and death rates and war losses. The population growth rate is, however, 1.5 percent annually now because of a declining natality rate and a fast-decreasing mortality rate. In 1961 the birth rate was 22.7 per 1,000 population. The rate of stillbirths was 82 per 1,000 born alive.

The population is predominantly engaged in agriculture and cattle raising, although the percentage of industrial workers and employees grows annually. In 1931, 76.6 percent of the population was engaged in agriculture; in 1948, 70.5 percent and in 1961, 50.6 percent.

In 1964 the average personal income was 37,000 dinars.* The standard of living is generally increasing with the improved effectiveness of production. The diminution of the average number in a household contributes to the increased standard of living, particularly in towns and industrial centers. In 1931, the average number of members of a household was 5.14. In 1953, it decreased to 4.29. In 1961 it was only 3.90. This decrease is especially noticeable among the more civilized parts of the population in the north and the west and especially in the towns. Although more of the population are now in towns than ever before, 59 percent of the population in 1961 lived in communities of 2,000 inhabitants or less. In 1961 there were only seven cities with over 50,000 inhabitants and six cities with over 100,000. Life in towns and industrial communities has brought about some radical change in employment, habitation, communication, and social relationships—for example, the increased number of women in the work force.

There has been a dramatic growth of education. Fifty-five percent of the population in 1921 was illiterate. In 1953 this number was decreased to 25.4 percent and in 1961 to 19.7 percent. Now most illiteracy occurs in obscure villages in the underdeveloped southeast. In 1961 there were over 9,000,000 persons with elementary educations, over 500,000 with secondary school educations, and over 200,000 with high school educations.

The sociopolitical system is codified by a series of democratically promulgated laws beginning from November 29, 1943, when new Yugoslavia was proclaimed, up to the present day. The basic sociopolitical aim of the country throughout this period has been the building of a humanistic-socialistic system. Its principles, in the present phase of development, are codified by the latest Constitution, that of April 7, 1963: social owner-

---

* In 1964, one dollar was equivalent to seven hundred and fifty dinars.

ship of the means of production; free congregation and self-government of the working people within the working organization and sociopolitical communities—the municipality, the district, the republic, and the federation; distribution from the working organizations according to labor performed in keeping with the principle "from each according to his abilities, to each according to his labor"; the achievement of democratic political relations through social management according to the system of elected representative bodies; and peaceful cooperation with all peoples in accordance with the principles of coexistence.[2]

The intensive industrialization and urbanization of this backward, agricultural country has been carried out in accordance with a series of principles of socialist economy. In the period 1945–1946 socioeconomic development was characterized by state control of many industrial and trade enterprises, by decreases in the private industrial and trade economy, and by maximizing control of the agricultural and artisan economies and the favoring of cooperative movement in them. 1947–1949 was a period of formation of heavy and light industry, intensive employment of the workers in industry and mining, and changes in the structure of population, followed by formation of industrial colonies and the enlargement of towns. In 1950–1953, because of the economic blockade and threats from the countries of the Eastern bloc, the economy was characterized by a decrease of industrial production of consumer goods, by the strengthening of war industry and the defensive power of the country, and by a decrease of employment and investment in the building industry. Since 1952, there has been an increase of industrial production; an increase of production of consumer goods; economic relations with the Western countries, the developing countries, and, in the last years, with Eastern countries; greater initiative by the producers and by the workers; self-management of enterprises; intensive urbanization and other changes in the ways of living, including raised standards; and a renewed favoring of private and collective agriculture and crafts and of economic management in businesses. In 1965, with the stabilization of currency,* a phase stressing overall economic reforms began. This involved Yugoslavia in the international distribution of labor, and meant increasing the number of direct producers and returning to intensive farming.

The favorable political and economic conditions made possible the development of an extensive and varied cultural life in contemporary Yugoslavia, particularly in towns and industrial settlements.

---

* One dollar is equivalent to 12.50 new dinars (or 12.50 old dinars).

Together with the general cultural progress, very satisfactory conditions have been created for health and social protection. In 1962 there were 2,996 health institutions and pharmacies. The total number of beds in stationary institutions amounted in that year to 100,360, i.e., 1 bed per 187 inhabitants. In the health institutions there worked 13,101 doctors, or 1 doctor per 1,437 inhabitants. In the same institutions there were 18,257 nurses and technicians or 1 nurse or technician per 1,031 inhabitants. There were 1,672 protective institutions for children and youth and 130 institutions for protection of adults with 8,694 persons, or 1 per 2,166 inhabitants, working in them.

It should be noted that all employees of social institutions as well as the members of their families have health and pension insurance from the contribution of enterprises and institutions and from the social-insurance fund. Such insurance is also provided for workers in private employment by the employers. Lastly, peasants, craftsmen, and other self-employed workers may have health protection, too, if they donate a specified contribution. Health insurance provides free ambulance service and use of stationary health institutions; free medical and sanitary supplies; free medical treatment; paid sick leave and maternity leave; paid expenses for the clothing of a newborn infant and expenses in the case of death; and an allowance for children. Pension insurance provides a personal or family pension for either age or disability, whether permanent or temporary.

In 1963 the total expenses of the social insurance service amounted to 15,376,000 dinars, i.e., about 850,000 dinars per person. Communal funds provide for uninsured social cases such as the unemployed, the disabled, invalids, the aged, and patients suffering from tuberculosis and venereal and chronic mental diseases. In 1962, the total expenses of social aid amounted to 4,824,000 dinars, i.e., about 250,000 dinars per inhabitant.[34, 39]

THE HISTORIC DEVELOPMENT OF PSYCHIATRY

History and culture conditioned the characteristic development of medicine in Yugoslavia. As V. Stanojevic has written:

The cultural factor, firmly connected with the geographical and racial factor, is trailed as a red thread throughout the whole of the past of Yugoslav peoples, giving to their culture—until the fall of the Roman Empire—a unique feature of the West, and after that fall and the invasion of Osmanli not only the feature of division of East and West but also the division into three religions: Orthodox, Roman Catholic, and Moslem, each of them introducing the features of its own culture: the Orthodox-Byzantine culture with its monastic hospitals and charitable institutions, as well as priests' prayers for the healing of the sick; the Roman Catholic—Western culture, in which the ecclesiastics and priests open hospitals, keep pharmacies, come into connection with similar institutions in Italy, Germany, and Hungary, cultivate medicinal herbs in monastery gardens, introduce into ecclesiastical books rules about health preservation and write popular medical books, and provide the monastery libraries with medical works in Latin; the Moslem-Arabic culture with its hygiene and dietetic regulations about drinking water and water supplies, fountains, and hammamums, and its medical aid from the Mohammedan priests who cured with amulets and prescriptions borrowed from the works of Arabic medical writers. Divided into geographic and religious cultural spheres, and having to borrow from neighboring cultural centers because of its backwardness, the medicine of Yugoslav peoples drew medical knowledge at the beginning and for centuries from constant agents and established sources: the eastern part through local ecclesiastical and learned men from Byzantium or through travelling foreign physicians, mostly of Greek or other Levantine nationality; the western part through Dubrovnik and other centers on the Adriatic coastline from Italy, where they acquired books and Italian doctors and pharmacists, educating later their own; the Moslem part through the Mohammedan priests and from Arabic medical sources. Although set apart by their agent sources, these three medical branches helped and complemented one another, and it was Dubrovnik that excelled in it most of all, which offered medical knowledge and gave medical services to the hinterland. With the transfer of cultural-medical centers from Italy to the west and after the fall of Byzantium, as well as after the formation of new medical centers in the north in the mid-eighteenth century in the form of "old Viennese medical schools," the basis for medical borrowings of all Yugoslav peoples is transferred to these parts. Having failed even by 1918 to form a permanent independent state and an independent medical culture by serving foreign national cultures Yugoslav peoples gave to other peoples a number of their famous and remarkable cultural workers, and among them many famous physicians.[35]

The development of psychiatric culture was defined within the framework of the development of medical and general culture. The apocryphal manuscripts about national saints and the monastic manuscripts describe the accommodation of mental patients in monastic hospitals in the early Middle Ages. As early as 1199, there was a hospital in the monastery of Hilandar on Mount Athos, and in 1208 a hospital was built in the monastery Studenica. Both were built by Saint Sava, also the founder of the Serbian Orthodox Church and the son of the founder of the Serbian state, Stephen Nemanja. The use of wooden shackles and exorcistic procedures in the treatment of the mentally ill can be seen on medieval frescoes in monasteries, and in old church manuscripts. Such therapy persists today in some monasteries in the Balkans, and in Macedonia, therapy by charms can still be found. The survival of folk medicine can also be observed in the eastern parts of the country.[5, 18, 37]

In the west of the country during the later medieval period strict decrees against sorcerers and pagan medicine were promulgated. Witches were prosecuted in accordance with the Inquisition. Then in 1740 the Austrian Czarina Maria Therezia forbid the execution of witches and in 1768 a law on juridicial and criminal proceedings distinguished mental illness from mental disturbances due to mystical agencies. A more realistic comprehension of the nature of diseases and treatment of patients began.

At that time the coastal areas were influenced by Italian medical centers and educated doctors concerned themselves with rules for the care of mental patients. Despite this, the handling of patients was not humane. They were often put into city towers and prisons and tied by chains. Mental illness was viewed as a penalty for their amoral behaviour or that of their family. Popular books (*lekarusa*) of the time included numerous prescriptions for the cure of mental patients by medicaments. Religious and mystical therapy was also found in the coastal regions, although less than in the eastern parts because of the influence of Roman Catholicism and Western medicine. Wealthier patients were often sent to asylums in Austria and Italy, and this influenced to some extent more optimistic attitudes toward mental illness. In Croatia, Slavonia, and Dalmatia, which were under Hungarian jurisdiction, treatment was more humane.

Humanistic reform in the understanding and treatment of mental patients developed in Yugoslavi countries during the nineteenth century. In 1804, a public hospital was founded in Zagreb, under the management of the Catholic Order of Charitable Brothers, and it had a department for the mentally ill in its courtyard. A lunatic asylum was founded in Zadar in 1807, as part of a public hospital, by the civil government for Dalmatia within the French empire. A government decree based on the humane principles of Pinel was issued. Several mental hospitals were founded shortly thereafter: at Ljubljana in 1811, at Dubrovnik in 1830, and at Rijeka in 1857. In 1856 after the stabilization of the Austro-Hungarian rule, the Governors' Council for Croatia, Dalmatia, and Slavonia issued some humane instructions for the reception, treatment, and dismissal of mental patients from lunatic departments in these areas. The instructions emphasized that patients could only be received with a doctor's testimony and the permission of the civil organ of the Governor's Council. It should be noted that lunatic departments at this time did not have physicians and only served to accommodate patients. However, humane reform of this type did not occur in the Balkans where religious, mystical, or popular medicine was still taking place in monasteries.[8, 10]

PSYCHIATRY

Professional psychiatry developed in the second half of the nineteenth century with the founding of mental hospitals managed by doctors, many of whom had trained in Austria, Germany, or France.

The first hospital for mental disease was founded in Belgrade, Serbia. In 1861, Prince Michael signed the official "Regulations on the Foundation of a Home for the Tusques" and ordained that the Asylum be settled in an adapted private house of the deceased court doctor, B. S. Kunibert (Kunibert's Tower). The "Home for the Mind's Descended" was inaugurated on August 26, 1861, and had twenty-five beds in all. Its chief and only doctor was Florian Bürg. Later, Mladen Jankovic, who had trained in Germany, introduced the use of medicinal therapy. Because of overcrowding, new buildings were built and by the end of the nineteenth century, there were some 200 to 250 patients annually. In 1881, Jovan Danic, who had trained in Paris, became head of the asylum and introduced the contemporary system of diagnosis, classification, therapy, and record keeping.[11, 28]

Experience in Belgrade influenced developments elsewhere. In 1877, an asylum for the Tusques was built in Zagreb, modeled after the Krafft-Ebing asylum in Gratz. A modern mental hospital with 250 beds was built in Stenjevac near Zabreb (now Vrapee) in 1879. Its first chief was Ivan Rôhacek. He was followed by Ivan Zirovcic.[9] This hospital soon proved to be too small to accommodate the 300 to 500 patients who passed through it annually. In 1883, an eighty-bed asylum was founded in Sibenik, Dalmatig, as an annex to the public hospital. Its first head was Aurel Zlatarevic, a specialist psychiatrist, educated in Gratz under Professor Krafft-Ebing. Similar mental hospitals were founded elsewhere under the Austro-Hungarian rule: in 1881, in Studenac, Slovenia, under the management of Karel Bleiweis-Trsteniski; in 1894 in Sarajevo, under C. Bayer; and in 1902 in Danilovgrad, under Jovan Kujacic.[8, 10, 28]

These institutions made possible professional and scientific psychiatric work such as that of J. Danic on alcoholism and mental disorders in Serbia, of A. Zlatarevic on statistical trends of mental illness in Dalmatia, and of I. Zirovcic on forensic psychopathology in Croatia and V. Subotic on some special forms of mental disorders in Serbia. Most important are the unwritten accomplishments by the pioneers of Yugoslav psychiatry which became part of the institutions in which they worked and into which they brought the principles and methods of world psychiatry of that time.[10, 26]

After the foundation of the Yugoslav state in 1918, psychiatry developed rapidly, but under the influence of neurology. Between the two world wars five mental hospitals were founded and old ones were reconstructed. However conditions were difficult. There was overcrowding, a small number of physicians, inadequately trained assistants, and insufficient funds.

A new phase in the development of Yugoslav psychiatry began with the opening of the neuropsychiatric clinics within the medical faculties of universities and the neuropsychiatric departments within public hospitals in Belgrade, Ljubljana, and Sarajevo. This led to the treatment of neurotics and the introduction of psychotherapy. In 1912, the Neurologic-Psychiatric Clinic was founded in Zagreb by Professor Mihajlo Lapinski and in 1932, Professor Radoslav Lopasic became its head. Since then it has been the main center for the development of contemporary principles and methods. In 1923, a neuropsychiatric clinic was founded in Belgrade by Professor Laza Stanojevic, who was himself mainly interested in contemporary biological methods. Beginning in 1920, lectures were given at the medical faculty in Ljubljana by Professor Alfred Serko, a disciple of Kraepelin and Wagner-Jauregg, who had experimented on himself with mescaline and had attended Freud's and Adler's courses. A major role was also played by independent sanitariums, in which psychoanalysis was adopted and developed together with other psychotherapeutic methods.[24]

In 1932, the Society of Yugoslav Psychiatrists was founded. It was instrumental in the organization of psychiatric service and national and international communication and in the development of professional and scientific work. The basic theoretical orientation of the Society was organic and biological with emphasis on the study of hereditary factors.

Also in 1932, some psychologically oriented psychiatrists founded the Yugoslav Society for Mental Hygiene, with special sections in Belgrade, Zagreb, and Ljubljana. It opposed the biological orientation and advocated psychological and social principles, therapy, and prevention.[23]

Although they participated in the activities of the Society for Mental Hygiene, some Belgrade psychoanalysts and other followers of psychoanalysis outside the circle of psychiatrists founded a Society for Psychoanalysis in Belgrade in 1938. Its leader, A. Sugar, was killed in a German concentration camp in World War II. This society organized translations, made popular the basic principles of psychoanalysis, and arranged for the training of other psychoanalysts. The members of that first and only Society for Psychoanalysis up to now were: A. Sugar, H. Klajn, V. Klajn, Lj. Dumic, Lj. Zivkovic, V. Matic, N. Popovic, M. Djuric, and V. Dvornikovic. The individual psychology of Adler was very much accepted at that time in some cultural and psychiatric circles and particularly by the Marxists, who attacked Freud's psychoanalysis from ideological positions. The psychoanalysts therefore were forced to become acquainted with Adler's ideas to better defend their own views in discussion. A more positive outlook on psychoanalysis in Yugoslavia has probably developed as a result of these efforts than was the case in some of the other East European countries, although other factors have certainly affected this phenomenon.

A new epoch in the development of Yugoslav psychiatry began after World War II. It was partly conditioned by an urgent need to repair psychiatric institutions damaged during the war, to compensate for the psychiatrists killed in the war, and to handle the mental problems worsened by the war. But the essential cause of the rapid development of psychiatry after the war consisted in the fundamental political, economic, and cultural transformation of Yugoslavia into a socialist country. The development of psychiatry corresponded with her progress.

In the first post-war period of restoration and construction and the formation of the so-called "administrative-socialistic system" the basic efforts were directed toward enlarging existent institutions and staffs as well as building new institutions in regions where they did not previously exist, as in Macedonia and Montenegro. In a number of general hospitals neuropsychiatric departments were founded. Finally neuropsychiatric clinics were founded at the new medical faculties in Ljubljana (1945), Sarajevo (1946), Skoplje (1947), and at the Military Medical Academy in Belgrade (1950).

According to the data of B. Niketic, in pre-war Yugoslavia there was a total of 5,200 psychiatric beds (including those in private sanatoriums). During the war a total of 1,495 beds were lost, so that immediately after the Liberation there were only 3,705 beds. By 1949 the yearly capacity of 6,149 beds was produced, and this already surpassed the pre-war capacity. According to the indexes given by D. Julius, in 1945, nineteen mental patients were hospitalized in Yugoslavia per 100,000 inhabitants; in 1950 the ratio was forty-five per 100,000. Since the need for psychiatric beds always surpassed the supply, the increase in beds could be generally explained by the increase in illness.[20]

But in this period the orientation remained predominantly biological-somatic. Special efforts were made toward the development of electroshock and insulin therapy. In psychotherapy the influences of Pavlov's or similar suggestive-persuasive methods predominated. In clinics and hospital wards the primacy of neurology continued and was reflected in an exclusive neuropathological trend in the investigation of psychiatric disorders. A very widespread theory at this time was V. Vujic's theory of larval encephalitis. Vujic explained the causes of a series of so-called "pseudo-neurasthenic" illnesses as originating in damage to the extrapyramidal system. This theory led to the application of a number of restrictive enforced working measures as treatment. Such a situation was rationalized with the assertion that a strict materialistic-organic orientation was being carried out, which assertion had really partly originated from the dogmatically understood Marxism of the Soviet school.

One of the basic consequences of the attitude was the denying of any scientism in psychodynamic theory and psychoanalytical therapy because they develop an unconscious mechanism. However, this antipsychological orientation resulted mostly from the retention of the classical ideas of German and French mechanistic-materialistic schools in which the bearers of the post-war psychiatry had been educated and which they then endeavored to proclaim as dialectical-materialistic. Because of that, in the Report on the State of Psychiatric Service in Yugoslavia given to the government of Yugoslavia in 1950 by Professors P. Lemkau and A. Pavkovic—the representatives to the World Health Organization—the following is concluded: a) there is an underdevelopment of psychodynamics and psychotherapy in the psychiatric practice and training; b) there is little collaboration between psychiatrists and subsidiary professionals, such as psychologists, social workers, therapists, and psychiatric nurses, and some of these professions do not exist; and c) there is a lack of practice and scientific work in the field of social psychiatry.

Apart from the observed deficiencies, these authors recommended immediate activity in the field of teaching psychiatry, a program of specialization in psychiatry, the formation of a center or an institute for collecting and elaborating data about mental illnesses, the establishment of inspecting and consulting services for psychiatristic institutions, and the education of the people in the field of mental hygiene. Another plan recommended sending psychiatrists for specialization into foreign centers, particularly for the fields of psychotherapy, child psychiatry, clinical psychology, psychiatric social services, and mental hygiene, and the improvement of the network of psychiatric hospitals and clinics.[23] In the first professional and scientific assemblies these latter recommendations provoked lively and very contrary discussions, and they were gradually realized.

The second period of post-war psychiatry was democratization, decentralization, and self-government. The abandonment of dogmatic, pseudo-Marxist ideas and the adoption of original Marxist theories and practices in the country has certainly played a great role in this. Finally, an enormous part in this renaissance has been played by the younger generation of psychiatrists and other medical and cultural experts, who spent time in medical and cultural centers of Europe and America or were familiar with professional literature from these countries.

In 1953 two institutions with psychodynamic orientations were founded. Within the Zagreb neuropsychiatric clinic Professor Stjepan Betlheim, educated in Vienna, founded a department for psychotherapy which was analytic or analytically oriented. In the same year Professor Vojin Matic of Belgrade, educated in Paris, founded a medical-psychological consulting institution (child guidance center) in which a working and educative center for child psychotherapy of an analytic type was formed. Although, unfortunately, this center stopped its activity after ten years, during that time it succeeded in introducing a series of new influences into Belgrade psychiatric institutions. In 1956, the psychotherapist Vladislav Klajn formed the neuropsychiatric department at the Dr. D. Misovic Hospital in Belgrade, which became a working and educative center for the psychotherapy of adults and for the therapy of psychosomatic disorders.

In the last ten years, the capacities and the variety of psychiatric institutions and staff have increased remarkably. Among other important institutes that opened were the new professional and educative centers within the medical faculties in Rijeka (1955), Novi Sad (1960), and Nis (1961), and the departments for psychopathology within the faculties of philosphy in Belgrade and Zagreb. In addition, a number of psychiatric departments have been opened within general hospitals, and various dispensaries and consulting institutions for mental health have been built in many large towns. The number of neuropsychiatrists is four times greater than it was ten years ago, and the number of people in psychiatry and its separate branches has similarly increased. Since subsidiary staffs are formed, teamwork is becoming more and more the rule. Particularly important is the progress achieved by the collaboration with hospital services that is developing more and more. In the hospital institutions, polymorphous ways of work and investigation have developed which comprise the neurophysiological as well as the psychosocial elements in the problems of mental disorders and the mentally ill.

However, the most important progress in Yugoslav psychiatry has, no doubt, been achieved in the field of its general philosophical orientation. Instead of a bio-organical positive orientation the holistic dynamic orientation predominates more and more, in which an integration of biological, psychological, and social elements in the field of causes, consequences, and possibilities of therapy and prevention is being attempted. Because of such an orientation it is not only practice which becomes modernized; the direction of psychiatric education is more and more changing, so that together with somatic and neurophysiological aspects, psychological and sociocultural aspects of theory and practice are taught as well. Because of that many "super specialties" are coming into being as are stronger aspirations for making psychiatry independent—by which this epoch of development will probably be crowned.

THE FREQUENCY OF MENTAL DISORDERS

Although the exact epidemiological data about the frequency of mental disorders in the country are not available as of now, rather clear conclusions can be drawn from the available data. The global frequency of mental disorders is constantly increasing, they occupy a more and more important place in the general morbidity, and they obtain more complex aspects of appearance. This results in more serious social consequences. The empirical observation of these facts by medical experts and social functionaries helped bring about the status of psychiatry as a science. On the other hand, the failure of biological therapy within exclusively hospital or dispensary practice, together with the increasing success of pioneer efforts in the field of psychosocial therapy, encouraged the rise of dynamic, psychosocial orientation in psychiatry and mental hygiene.

According to M. Kilibarda's estimated data received on the basis of data from the Federal Institute for Public Health about diagnoses at first examinations in the dispensary and clinical institution and other sources, the morbidity of mental disorders in Yugoslavia is shown by Tables 1–4.[31, 38]

TABLE 1.

The Increase of Mental Disorders in Yugoslavia, 1950–1964.

Year	Number	Percent of total morbidity	Rate per 1,000 inhabitants
1950	65,784	0.63	4.05
1951	78,019	0.78	4.70
1952	98,244	0.97	5.85
1953	129,539	1.15	7.60
1954	168,502	1.33	9.75
1955	191,197	1.39	10.91
1956	194,220	1.36	10.98
1957	223,213	1.35	12.50
1958	280,975	1.62	15.59
1959	332,428	1.67	18.25
1960	453,477	1.88	24.64
1961	633,413	2.47	34.04
1962	723,826	2.69	38.43
1963	765,590	2.93	40.20
1964	864,280	3.08	44.10

On the basis of the data from Table 1, it is easily observed that the number of disorders in 1950–1964 increased 13.1 times, that their participation in general morbidity increased 4.9 times, and that the rate of mental disorders increased 10.7 times. It can be reasonably supposed that a great number of mentally diseased, and particularly those from underdeveloped

TABLE 2.

The Morbidity of Mental Disorders with the Socially Insured, 1952–1964.

Year	Number	Percent of total morbidity	Rate per 1,000 inhabitants
1952	62,903	1.05	34.8
1953	75,492	1.18	38.2
1954	96,963	1.40	43.3
1955	82,415	1.40	33.2
1956	108,438	1.41	43.2
1957	121,813	1.23	48.3
1958	153,363	1.70	50.7
1959	178,905	1.75	55.6
1960	242,920	2.03	69.8
1961	324,743	2.58	89.0
1962	371,155	2.83	116.3
1963	378,644	3.07	99.0
1964	400,524	3.05	97.8

areas, did not ask for medical aid—not at least for psychiatric aid. Because of that the quoted data are insufficient. Thus, the survey of the rate of mental disorders with those employed in state services, who have social insurance and better possibilities for asking and using the specialist doctor's aid, are more instructive.

It can be clearly seen that the rate of illness in Table 2 is far greater than that in the previous one. But, here the number of illnesses has increased 6.3 times, its importance in the general structure of morbidity is increased 2.9 times, and the prevalence has increased about 3 times. Between 1953 and 1962, because of greater treatment facilities, the prevalence rate of mental disorders increased differently in separate Socialistic Republics, as shown in Table 3.

TABLE 3.

The Rate of Mental Disorders with the Socially Insured in Socialist Republics per 1,000 Inhabitants in 1953 and 1964.

Year	SFRY	Serbia	Croatia	Slovenia	Bosnia and Herzegovina	Macedonia	Montenegro
1953	38.2	55.7	51.4	7.2	19.1	16.7	6.4
1964	97.8	149.9	74.3	41.8	42.3	109.6	98.1

The data in Table 3 show the particularly important increase of mental disorders in areas which experienced rapid changes in their structure because of industrialization and urbanization, especially Macedonia, Montenegro, and Serbia.

The data from Table 4 indicate clearly that the state of mental health is indeed becoming more and more seriously disordered in the whole country. These suicide rates put Yugoslavia in the upper half of the world's list according to suicide frequency. Highly industrialized areas of Slovenia and Vojvodina have especially high suicide rates.[4, 27]

The increasing importance of mental disorders in the country is shown by the available data about their social consequences. The number of sick leaves per 1,000 of the insured has increased sevenfold in the period from 1952 to 1961, while the number of lost working days increased over 5 times. In the same year the patients with mental disorders occupied, besides that, 3.35 percent of the total number of temporary working disabilities, while their participation in the pensioning because of illness amounted to 6.7 percent. According to informal data from the social insurance service, these indicators are increasing from year to year.[6]

TABLE 4.

Suicide per 100,000 Inhabitants in Socialistic Republics and Provinces of Yugoslavia, 1953–1963.

Year	Yugo-slavia	Serbia				Croatia	Slovenia	Bosnia and Herzo-govina	Mace-donia	Monte-negro
		Total	Proper	Vojvo-dina	Kosovo-Medohia					
1953	9.7	10.7	9.6	17.1	2.9	11.2	19.7	5.0	2.5	13.5
1954	10.7	11.0	9.5	18.5	3.4	12.3	23.2	5.0	2.6	16.0
1955	11.0	10.9	9.0	19.7	3.3	13.1	22.8	5.6	2.5	10.6
1956	10.5	10.4	8.7	18.0	3.8	12.3	22.4	5.7	2.8	11.4
1957	11.2	11.5	9.7	20.7	2.5	12.8	22.8	6.2	2.9	13.4
1958	10.9	10.9	9.0	20.2	2.1	12.6	23.6	5.7	3.1	13.9
1959	12.1	11.3	9.5	20.2	3.3	12.5	25.8	7.4	3.1	13.7
1960	11.9	11.5	9.8	20.8	2.4	14.6	25.5	7.2	3.5	13.0
1961	12.0	12.0	10.0	21.0	4.0	15.0	23.0	7.0	3.0	13.0
1962	13.1	12.9	11.3	22.6	2.2	14.8	29.0	6.8	5.1	14.5
1963	12.8	12.7	10.6	23.4	3.5	14.6	28.3	7.8	3.9	11.2

The data from epidemiological surveys in two factories in Montene-gro, the fastest changing region in the country, should be mentioned. In the "Tik" textile factory in Titograd, it was found that 46.2% of the employees (40.6% males and 47.8% females) had mental disorders. In the "Rudes" paper factory in Ivangrad, it was found that 19.4% (18.1% males, 24.8% females) had mental disorders.[15] These data confirm certain clinical epidemiological suppositions, and emphasize the increase of neu-rotic disorders in the face of socio-cultural changes in the country.

According to the data of mental hospitals, the greatest number of patients were between 30 and 39 years of age. The number of patients increases gradually, starting in the age group 20–29 years, and reaches the maximum in the age group 30–39 years. It gradually declines in the next age groups. According to the data of psychiatric clinics and departments, the greatest frequency is also in the age group 30–39 years of age, for both sexes, and related data are similar. In all age groups, the number of women patients predominates.

Over 60 percent of patients stayed more than five years in mental hospitals; 24.5 per cent were hospitalized up to six months. In the psy-chiatric clinics and departments the average length of hospitalization for psychosis was 126 days, for psychoneurosis, 28 days, for disorder of character and intelligence, 134 days.

The frequency distribution of specific types of mental disorders essentially corresponds to patterns found in other countries, with schizo-phrenic psychoses accounting for the largest number of cases.[25] If the data on the distribution of frequency of mental disorders are correlated with the available epidemiological data from the rest of the world, then certain tentative conclusions can be drawn. The extent of psychiatric disorders in Yugoslavia represents a position between highly developed cultures (with more complicated neuroses, sociopathic, functional psy-chotic disorders) and underdeveloped cultures (with more expressed organic–psychotic, and primitive, neurotic disorders). In Yugoslavia, these differences can be observed in respect to the qualititative state of psy-chiatric morbidity in western and eastern parts of the country.[3, 15-19, 36]

POSITION AND PRINCIPLES OF PSYCHIATRY

In the last ten years there has been an ever-increasing interest in psychiatry, not only in terms of new hospital programs and the numbers of physicians deciding on careers in psychiatry, but also on the part of the general public. However, there still exist medical circles—including neuropsychiatrists—as well as social scientific circles, that are against psychiatry. Using various obsolete theories and prejudices they speculate on the very subject and practicability of psychiatry or even on the knowledge of mental health. Some medical circles attack psychiatry in the name of materialistic and biophysical medicine, to which a more developed neurology would be much closer. These attacks result mainly from inadequate knowledge of psychology and social science. More important are the objections of those who underestimate the importance of psychiatric disturbances and who claim that these are merely so-called "organic disturbances" of mental life. Some eminent representatives of society and social-scientific circles claim that psychiatric disorders are characteristics of decadent societies, or societies with class and economic conflicts, and therefore they are of no importance in Yugoslavia. Some intellectual circles have developed contradictory theories which claim that the entire industrial and urban development of the country with the current modern culture is an expression of human estrangement from its essential nature. Therefore, they have magnified the importance and practicability of psychiatry making it a kind of social science and practice.

Although the basic characteristic of the new psychiatric theory is pluralistic, there is a tendency toward integration and uniformity, especially within individual psychiatric centers. Classical organic psychiatry is still very strong in Yugoslavia. It dominates the academic orientations of departments of psychiatry at medical faculties, with the exception of Zagreb. Still, a pure organic conception hardly exists (as it did after World War II, when the majority of neurotic disorders were explained by symptomatology of the larval encephalitis or similar inflamations or intoxications of the central nervous system) but it is combined and interlaced with dynamic conceptions. Within dominating organologic conceptions a minor part is taken by the principles of the constitutionalistic school, although they have largely survived in the field of the so-called "endogenetic" psychosis and partly in the so-called "psychopathy." More important are the principles of reflexological theory, particularly in the field of neurosis. Still, the most important conceptions are somatologic for the principles of diagnostics and therapy as well as for the direction of research and interpretation of their results. Such conceptions generally maintain the supremacy of neurology over psychiatry, although a number of concessions will be given to psychiatry and its practice.

It is clear also that dynamic conceptions continue to arise in Yugoslav psychiatry. However, they have not up to now become exclusive in any clinic or other psychiatric center or institution. Within dynamic psychiatry is a certain amount of heterogeneity. Pure psychoanalytic theory is being developed only within the Psychotherapeutic Department of the Neuropsychiatric Clinic in Zagreb. But even in that department there are tendencies toward and implications of certain theoretical corrections, emanating from the field of culture and social science. Far more developed are neo-analytic trends, particularly K. Horney's and E. Fromm's at the Neuropsychiatric departments in the Dr. D. Misovic Hospital in Belgrade. Besides those, there are significant influences of the German psychodynamic schools of E. Kretschmer and Schulz, particularly at the psychotherapeutic department of the psychiatric clinic in Ljubljana. Recently, principles of community psychiatric trends, after the school of M. Jones and J. Bierer, have also been successfully developed, particularly at the Institute for Mental Health in Belgrade, but so are some modern psychiatric hospitals in Vrapce, Belgrade, and Kovin and a number of non-hospital institutions.

The confrontation of organologic and dynamic trends leads more and more to a specific theoretical integration. Some experts individually adopt certain holistic principles and in some institutions there develops a coexistence between those who pursue different trends, with mutual influences and concessions. In this way, neuropsychiatry became connected with different branches of organic medicine, neuropathology, and neurophysiology on the one hand, and with psychology, humanistic disciplines, and social sciences on the other. Owing to all this, organic and dynamic psychiatry have developed simultaneously. Finally, psychiatry has started to influence medicine towards adopting principles of psychosomatic medicine and the sociology of medical institutions. At the same time the influence of modern psychiatry is felt in various institutions concerned with social problems and mental health.

LEGISLATION AND ORGANIZATION OF PSYCHIATRIC SERVICE

The uniform organization of psychiatric service is defined by the General Health Protection and Health Service Law of 1964, on the basis of which are made regulations for various health institutions and services. According to this law, medical institutions and medical staff are directly in charge of health service. Medical institutions can be of various types:

polyclinics, dispensaries, hospitals, boards of health, etc. They function as independent institutions with self-management. Various sociopolitical institutions as well as some individual citizens take part in the management of them. All medical institutions under municipal, district, republic, and federation administration are united into a system of health centers which coordinate in the formation of their programs and organize medical service in their territories. Health centers function under the principles of self-management and social self-government, like all other medical institutions. They are localized within the framework of a well-developed medical institution in a sociopolitical unit. Each sociopolitical unit assures suitable conditions for the activity of these institutions in its territory. Sociopolitical units are, according to the Constitution, represented by elected social and administrative bodies and executive governments which are arranged hierarchically. Although major bodies can only partly give orders to the minor ones, they direct and control them.

According to the Constitution all citizens are entitled to health insurance. They can choose medical institutions and physicians. Persons who are socially insured—those who are employed in social services, or those who are not but pay regularly for their insurance—are entitled to get free medical treatment, whereas citizens who are not insured pay for the medical services themselves. In special cases the medical treatment of those not insured is paid by the sociopolitical unit (according to regulations, psychotic mental patients are freed from paying for their treatment). Besides that, preventive medicine is financed from the funds of the sociopolitical units. According to law, medical staffs are self-reliant and independent in their work, but are responsible for it. They cannot practice privately, although special regulations allow private practice under certain conditions (e.g., retired physicians, or those in regions lacking medical staff). It is very important to stress that there is a general tendency to localize health service within municipalities and so-called "communes," which are basic economic and political units in a territory under the administration of a municipal assembly, and to establish and develop independent health centers.[7]

Organizational schemes, plans, and programs of the health centers include the promotion of mental health services, according to the propositions of the World Health Organization. Therefore, health centers, particularly those in communes, functionally integrate psychiatric and other institutions concerned with problems of mental health (curing, rehabilitation, and prevention). They make plans and programs for the development of such institutions and for the specialization of the professional staffs who work in them (doctors, psychiatrists, nurses, psychologists, social workers, and work therapists). Commissions for mental health have been formed within health centers in various communes and republics and in the federations which coordinate psychiatric and mental health work in their territories. According to information given by N. Persic and P. Korporic, in the Socialist Republic of Croatia, where psychiatric service is better organized than anywhere else in the country, the complex organization of mental health protection functions at present in the following way: Main responsibility is with dispensaries for mental health protection; these dispensaries are divisions of the health centers, i.e., psychiatric clinics or neuropsychiatric departments. According to their practicability and tasks, dispensaries are formed within municipalities, districts, and republics. Together with hospitals, dispensaries are responsible for mental health protection in their territory. Because they are structurally differentiated, however, the territory and range of their work are greater. Thus, for example, the Central Dispensary, besides its practice, has the educative role within that republic. Dispensaries can be concerned with general psychiatric service or specialized ones.

Hospitals and other psychiatric institutions—mental hospitals, neuropsychiatric departments and clinics for psychotherapy, rehabilitation, mental defectives, and delinquents—have developed wider ranges of activities. Firstly, they have integrated curative and preventive aspects of psychiatric work. Then, they have become functionally connected with nonhospital institutions, either within themselves or within their health center. Some have even become organizational units of a health center. Some have become organizational units of educative centers in cases where there were no possibilities for localization of organizational units of health centers or nonhospital institutions of the dispensary type. Some hospitals specialize, whereas in others various functional centers are formed: centers for active therapy, working therapy, curing of alcoholics, epileptics, and delinquents. However, there is a general tendency, in all such institutions, toward developing dispensary-type departments which would mediate between hospitals and the society. Finally, there are more and more neuropsychiatric departments formed within hospitals and organized on the same principle of arrangement according to the territorial network.[31]

The greatest progress has been achieved in the development and organization of mental hospitals, neuropsychiatric departments of hospitals, and neuropsychiatric clinics. In Yugoslavia in 1945, there were only 0.19

beds for mental patients per 1,000 inhabitants, in 1950 there were 0.45 beds, in 1963 there were 0.67 beds. This nevertheless puts Yugoslavia among the last countries on the European list, among those which are under the minimum of 1 bed per 1,000 inhabitants, which is advised by the World Health Organization. The 12,691 psychiatric beds are only 12.1 percent of the total number of patients' beds in the country. However there exist considerable variations of the index of psychiatric beds found among the socialistic republics (per 1,000 inhabitants): Croatia, 1.16; Slovenia, 1.13; Serbia, 0.53; Macedonia, 0.53; Montenegro, 0.40; and Bosnia and Herzegovina, 0.25. It should be added that the territorial distribution of beds is not in accord with the demographic distribution but with the state of development of corresponding health centers.

Of the total 12,691 psychiatric beds, 9,211 or 72.5 percent are in mental hospitals. This is 8.9 percent of the total number of beds in the country. Neuropsychiatric departments and clinics possess only 3,480 beds or 27.5 percent of the total psychiatric beds. This is 3.4 percent of the total number of hospital beds in the country. These data clearly show how overcrowded psychiatric institutions are, particularly in the backward parts of the country, and how difficult working is in these conditions.

In Serbia ten percent more patients are accepted per annum in hospitals than there are beds for them, and many more simply cannot be accepted. Thus the situation is similar to the one described above, in the section on the development of psychiatric hospitals in the country. However, the average number of days spent in mental hospitals in the period between 1952 and 1963 decreased from 493 to 345, and consequently, the holding power of hospitals partly increased. This development was caused by modern psychopharmaceutical means as well as sociotherapeutic and rehabilitation activities. Psychiatric service is best in neuropsychiatric departments and clinics, as patients spend less time there and are treated more as outpatients, which makes up for the lack of beds. In addition, in psychiatric departments and clinics psychiatric service is more complete; for example, at the neuropsychiatric clinic in Zagreb, there are the following departments: neurologic and psychiatric departments (for male and female), a psychotherapeutic department, a department for epilepsy, a neuropsychologic laboratory, a laboratory for biochemistry, a hematologic laboratory, and a photolaboratory. Besides, the clinic provides a well organized department for outpatients of a dispensary type, which is connected with other polyclinical services and the health service of the Zagreb Commune. At present the only psychiatric clinic separated from the neurologic clinic is the one in Ljubljana; at other clinics or departments these two activities are only partly divided, which affects the functional development of the psychiatric service.

The Federal Commission for Mental Health has found that for advice and directions, the outhospital psychiatric service is underdeveloped, even less developed than the one in hospitals and clinics. Many psychiatric hospitals, neuropsychiatric departments and clinics have not at all organized outhospital and dispensary service but only polyclinic and outpatient activities, which in fact only examine patients. Very often the outhospital service in health centers adopts the same system. Persic and Koporcic have found that in ten towns in Croatia, in psychiatric clinics for outpatients which are within health centers, there are approximately one or two doctors who are not permanently employed and work approximately two or three hours a day.[31] In all clinics neurological and psychiatric patients are examined together, which makes the situation even more difficult, as the examinations are directed more toward the neurologic type.

In bigger health centers, however, a real out-of-hospital and dispensary mental health service has developed. In Zagreb, Ljubljana, and Belgrade, large and well-organized dispensaries for mental hygiene, i.e., institutes for mental health, have been instituted which integrate preventive, therapeutic, and rehabilitative services. For example, the Belgrade Institute for Mental Health has the following departments: an open psychiatric department, a social rehabilitation department, a department for children and the young, and a scientific research department. In addition, there have been instituted smaller dispensaries in some large towns in the country, particularly in Croatia and Slovenia. In several towns there have also been established special dispensaries for alcoholics, epileptics, and juvenile delinquents. A number of neuropsychiatric departments of hospitals and some psychiatric hospitals have organized collaboration between their outpatient service, working on a dispensary basis, and the institutions for social and health protection in their territory.

Within the integrated service of health protection, the activities of mental hygiene function in the framework of specialized health protection. Such are dispensaries for pregnant women (in 1962 there were 560 such institutions), dispensaries for infants and school children (in 1962 there were 317), medical and psychological dispensaries and children's outpatient clinics (in 1962 there were 365). Apart from that, mental hygiene and psychiatric services function in institutions for social protection: in welfare centers, in communes, in orphanages (in 1962, there were 1,661 such institutions), in homes for poor children (in 1962 there were 31), in the old people's homes (in 1962 there were 130).

Psychiatric and mental health service is connected with educational institutions, particularly those concerned with mentally defective children. In Yugoslavia, in 1962, there were fifteen institutions for subnormal children in which 1,980 children lived (out of 2,335 found at the examination of school children). In 229 special departments and vocational schools there were 10,262 mentally backward children (out of 11,223). Psychiatric and mental health service is also becoming more closely connected with the service for rehabilitation of the physically defective, especially within the institutes for rehabilitation and physiotherapy.

This service is also connected with institutions concerned with delinquents, although as yet there are no social centers for treatment and rehabilitation of mentally defected delinquents and only in a few hospitals are there special departments for aggressive delinquents. But these activities are particularly significant in institutions for juvenile delinquents. [12, 16, 22, 29]

STAFF, PRACTICE, TEACHING, AND TRAINING IN PSYCHIATRY

The Federal Commission for Mental Health found in 1965 that the staff situation in psychiatry had improved quantitatively and qualitatively, but still was not satisfactory. According to the data given by D. Julius, in 1950, the situation in mental hospitals was as follows: These were 141 patients to 1 doctor, 1,018 patients to 1 nurse, 5.3 patients to 1 member of the staff.

The distribution of psychiatric beds as well as the distribution of the staff is not proportionally set in separate republics, so that the situation in the developed republics in this respect is better than in the underdeveloped republics. It should be mentioned, in addition, that the situation of medical staffs in Yugoslavia is relatively good compared to other European countries (1,200 inhabitants per 1 doctor). But the situation of psychiatric staffs is much worse (52,000 inhabitants to 1 neuropsychiatrist).[12]

In the polyclinic and dispensary service of the Republic of Croatia, there are only ten or twelve neuropsychiatrists permanently employed. Within the Republic the neuropsychiatrists are unevenly distributed: whereas in Zagreb there are 12,000 inhabitants to 1 neuropsychiatrist, in the health centers of the country there are between 40,000 and 350,000 inhabitants to 1 psychiatrist. Although Croatia is the most advanced republic in regard to psychiatric service, it is only recently that experts of other descriptions have begun to emerge and contribute more visibly to activities in this field, thus making for greater diversification.[31]

The socialized health protection service is the reason why such practice is carried only in social institutions and why there is practically no private practice. The normal working day in institutions is six hours, whereas in stationary institutions there exist additional twenty-four-hour tours of duty followed by one day off. In addition to Sundays and holidays, those employed in the psychiatric service are entitled to one six-week leave a year; one part of it is taken in summer and the other in winter. Owing to shortages of personnel, large numbers of patients, and the need for additional income, almost all psychiatrists and their associates put in many hours of part-time work in polyclinic-dispensary or social welfare institutions. It logically follows that their overwork affects their very efficiency.

At present, polyclinics meet the needs of routine work along with the constantly increasing number of patients. In view of this, and because of insufficient personnel and the prevailing orientation of doctors toward neurology, these institutions are confined to classification of patients and urgent therapy. Pharmacological treatment alone is practiced there, although the staffs also authorize sick leaves and send patients home or to psychiatric institutions of a higher degree as required. There are, however, several dispensaries where activities are better organized and more complex. Two examples are the Institution for Mental Health in Belgrade and the Central Dispensary for Mental Hygiene in Zagreb. These representative institutions have entirely integrated curative, rehabilitation, and prevention practices. In addition to pharmaceutic therapy, these institutions also engage in complex depth psychotherapy, social therapy (covering occupational therapy, therapy through play, group therapy, communal therapy and therapeutic clubs, day and night hospitals, and family and work environment manipulation). Such complex activities are carried on in dispensaries for alcoholics in Belgrade and Zagreb as well as in certain dispensaries for delinquent children and adolescents in Belgrade, Zagreb, and Ljubljana.

Psychiatry courses in Yugoslav medical schools only partially follow the same pattern, mostly in regard to the quantity of material. As for quality, there are great differences between the east and the west of the country. Courses in psychiatry are combined with those in neurology to form a single course in neuropsychiatry, as is the case in most other European countries. The total number of hours required in psychiatry classes and the total number of hours spent on practical exercises amount to fifty-eight each, which is obviously insufficient. However, this seems to be the case in most European universities, as can be seen in a report of the World Health Organization dealing with this matter.[1] Instruction in psychiatry can therefore be improved only by the introduction of a number of complementary noncompulsory classes in psychiatry and allied sciences. This has been done in Zagreb and Ljubljana, for instance, so that the total number of classes exceeds 100. The situation is brighter at certain humanist faculties. At the Faculty of Philosophy in Belgrade, for example, students of psychology, especially those specializing in clinical psychology, have about 300 class hours in psychopathology, clinical psychology, and mental hygiene, whereas students of sociology have as many social-psychiatry classes and exercises as the number of psychology classes which are offered at the Faculty of Medicine.

The curriculum depends on the orientation of the different departments. In Belgrade, there are twenty classes in descriptive psychopathology, twelve in general psychiatry, sixteen in clinical psychiatry (four of these in neurosis and twelve in psychosis), and ten in mental hygiene and social psychiatry. In Zagreb, where instruction is more complex, one half of the compulsory fifty-eight classes are in depth psychology, neurosis, and psychosomatic disorders, and the remainder deals with general psychiatry and psychosis. In addition to this, there are as many non-compulsory classes in medical psychology with psychotherapy and in mental hygiene with social psychiatry. The rest of the medical faculties in the western part of the country more or less adhere to the same program.

Due to the large number of students, the shortage of assistants and professors, and the insufficient number of classes, the training exercises are merely demonstrations of patients and explanations of treatment methods. It is only the more eager students who can have practical training tours of psychiatric centers which are particularly helpful to their knowledge of psychodiagnostics and psychotherapy. The situation has been somewhat improved with the opening of instruction centers in appropriate medical institutions outside their faculties of medicine. Postgraduate courses were introduced at the faculties of medicine two years ago, as well as at the faculties of philosophy, regarding clinical psychology and social psychiatry. Such courses facilitate professional improvement of psychiatrists and general practitioners in the field of mental health.[13, 14]

Specialization in neuropsychiatry is undertaken according to a set of regulations applicable throughout the country. Graduates from a faculty of medicine desirous of specializing in the field of neuropsychiatry must have one year as hospital interns and three years of practical work in medical institutions. They are also required to pass a special examination.

Training in analytical psychotherapy is carried on at those psychotherapeutic centers mentioned above. Classical training can only be received during studies abroad; doctors so specialized carry on their practice in institutions of general psychiatry. During specialization doctors perform under supervision their regular work for which they are normally paid. However, there are possibilities for voluntary specialization during which one is not paid if the institution in question is short of adequate funds and no social organization finances the program. The training is supplemented by various courses and seminars and by study of professional literature. There exist in the country only two psychiatry textbooks, plus several related manuals. Moreover, an adequate amount of basic literature has been translated into national languages, although most students speak at least one of the major world languages.

RESEARCH WORK IN PSYCHIATRY

There are numerous shortcomings in Yugoslav psychiatric research, primarily due to insufficient organization and lack of coordination in methodology. Measures have been taken over the last two or three years to organize research work to a greater extent, and to allocate adequate funds for it.

Work on problems of clinical psychology, describing somatic causes of mental disorders and the possibilities of their somatic treatment, is by far the most numerous. J. Glaser collected seventy-one publications on research in Yugoslavia and submitted these to the Second World Congress of Psychiatrists which was devoted to schizophrenia. The majority of these publications dealt with the hereditary or the somatic aspect of this mental disorder. The toxic, infectious, and endocrinological causes of mental disorders have also been dealt with exhaustively. Very important in this context are the works by the late V. Vujic's Belgrade School dealing with the psychiatric effects of the so-called "larvated encephalitis," as well as those on the various possibilities of clinical-neurological diagnosis of such states. The same problems have been dealt with in a far more complex manner by the Zagreb School of R. Lopasic and his associates. R. Lopasic has recently been engaged as a pioneer in clinical research on geriatric problems in psychiatry. The Zagreb School has very often examined other biological possibilities of the causality and treatment of mental disorders. Since there are numerous studies in pharmacotherapy, in the last congress a symposium was held on these problems, organized by N. Bohacek. One must not omit the very well-documented experimental-clinic works by N. Persic and his associates relating to the biochemical background of functional psychosis. Also worthy of mention is the work of M. Borstnar and his associates in Ljubljana who examined combined pharmacological-reflexological methods of treating mental disorders, with certain original modifications. Particular emphasis in this context ought to be given the significant examinations of somatic-psychological and reflexological type, conducted in industrial psychiatry by M. Savicevic and his associates.

Immediately after the war, the veterans of Yugoslav psychoanalysis, H. Klajn and S. Betlheim, published studies on war neurosis in *Partizans,* thus contributing to the development of contemporary psychoanalysis. Whereas H. Klajn later turned to the theatre and published works only on the psychoanalytic interpretation of art, S. Betlheim continued his intense research in the domain of psychoanalytical theory and practice and formed a research center with his associate, Professor D. Blazevic. Very soon new names emerged: V. Matic began publishing studies on psychoanalytical theory, therapy, and prevention as applied to disorders in children and adolescents and formed a research center with his associates. V. Klajn attempted a synthesis of the practical need for fast therapeutic work and the principles of dynamic psychiatry. In his monograph on neurosis he tried to find contact points between psychodynamic theory and reflexology, and between the principles of psychodynamic theory and dialectical materialism. L. Milcinski studied the problems of integration of bionomic psychotherapy and social therapy and arrived at some strikingly original solutions. Works in the fields of dynamic theory and practice in psychiatry were growing more numerous. This made it possible for S. Betlheim to organize, within the national congress held in 1964, a symposium on psychotherapy at which scientific achievements in this field were discussed.

Research in social psychiatry and mental hygiene are at the moment still in the initial stage of development, although the authors who studied problems of psychotherapy also dealt with certain problems of mental hygiene. The research of the late D. Julius on the organization of psychiatric services, emphasizing social therapeutics, ended with his un--timely death. B. Svecenski in the Yugoslav Army conducted significant research in the field of social psychiatry, particularly on sociopathy and suicide. N. Persic, together with P. Koporcic, made a very careful study of problems concerning the organization of psychiatric service in Yugoslavia on an up-to-date basis. His studies are now becoming a basis for further activities in that direction. One of the first champions and research workers in social psychiatry was J. Kanoni, who read a paper—a pioneer work—on that subject before a convention of neurologists and psychiatrists in 1956. The social problems arising from alcoholism and the organization of social therapy were the subject of many experts, notably Professor S. Stojiljkovic in Belgrade and V. Hudolin in Zagreb. Finally, the late M. Bedenic wrote the original handbook on problems of mental hygiene, based on personal experience in Croatia.

It must be said that little research has been done in Yugoslavia in the field of social-cultural psychiatry and psychiatric sociology. V. Jakovljevic has worked intensely in this field since 1953, focusing his interest on the sociogenetic, sociotherapeutic, and transcultural types of research. In addition to this, the same author is studying social-pathological problems which have not previously been studied in Yugoslavia. Organized epidemiological research has been conducted only partially. The pioneer research work carried out by R. Lopasic and his associates on the Island of Susak comes to mind most readily; however, the group's work remained, for the most part, in the field of genetics. M. Kilibarda formulated numerous epidemiological suppositions based on the available data supplied by the Health Service. P. Lemkau, with his Yugoslavian colleagues of Zagreb and Rijeka, conducted certain epidemiological examinations in Istria, a region of Yugoslavia. A group of authors* studied comparatively the impact of industrialization on mental health on a sample of the sociocultural circle examined. However, no significant attempt at systematic epidemiological research has yet been made. The Federal Commission for Mental Health, therefore, views the organization of epidemiological surveys of mental disorders as one of the most urgent needs of scientific work. Finally, there is evidence in recent years of a general theoretical approach

---

* M. Savcicevic, V. Jakovljevic, M. Kilibarda and their associates.

to mental health research which has been influenced by theories on the relationship between the individual and society, particularly the Marxist theory on man's nature and alienation. This research is based on the accumulated experience of philosophers, sociologists, and psychiatrists.[30, 32]

PERSPECTIVES FOR THE DEVELOPMENT OF YUGOSLAVIAN PSYCHIATRY

In view of the present situation, the perspectives for the development of psychiatry in Yugoslavia seem very bright. Such a statement can be made on the basis of the following facts: the awareness of the greater importance of science in mental health, the more intensive inclusion of psychiatric services in the system of health protection for the people, and the extension of the scope and content of psychiatric theory and practice. In addition, the development of psychiatry is stimulated by contemporary scientific currents in the world, on the one hand, and the humanistic and socialistic system of the country on the other hand.

The immediate expectations for development may best be evaluated through the survey of recommendations which were executed for the Social and Health Council of the Federal Assembly by the Federal Commission for Mental Health. These recommendations were made on the basis of careful analysis of the present situation and thus represent the most accurate appraisal of the state of Yugoslavian psychiatry.

Before quoting the recommendations, it is necessary to observe that they could be comprehended as law. However, in accordance with the social system of the country, which incorporates self-government, various health and social-political institutions, and collectives, only guidelines are offered. These guidelines are then implemented by the local institutions and collectives. Because of that, the further development of psychiatry will probably be for a certain time heterogeneous, according to the socio-cultural development of the corresponding social environments. But rational direction will undoubtedly lead to the increased homogenization of progress, so that the undertaken efforts will not be in vain.

The Federal Commission for Mental Health in 1965 executed the following recommendations:

1. It is necessary to immediately increase the bed capacity for bedridden patients, for all cases, both serious and light. Bed capacity represents the material base for the stationary protection of mental health. It can be seen from the data that our present bed capacity is low compared to that of other

European countries. If the fact that the number of out-hospital psychiatric institutions is very small should be added, then a clearer picture of the urgent need for the increase of bed capacity is obtained. As a minimum, 1 bed per 1,000 inhabitants should be provided, which means that it is necessary to provide an additional 6,300 beds. The quoted rate is less than half the rate which is accepted and performed in a number of European countries.

Bed capacity should be realized in the following ways: (a) the redistribution and increase of the capacity of some of the existing institutions, which are responsible for it in proportion to their size; (b) the opening of new psychiatric hospitals with a capacity of 300 to 500 beds, which should be formed in the medical centers according to the defined regional order; (c) the increase of bed capacity of the neuropsychiatric departments of general hospitals and neuropsychiatric clinics by increasing the capacity of the existing departments and clinics and by opening new ones in the hospitals where they do not exist; the neuropsychiatric departments and clinics are to provide at least fifteen percent of the hospital bed capacity: ten percent for psychiatric and five percent for neurologic patients.

Together with the enumerated institutions for psychiatric hospital protection it is necessary to establish specialized stationary institutions for the treatment and prevention of mental disorders as follows: (a) social and rehabilitational institutions of differentiated types which should serve as the intermediate institutions between hospitalization and the complete rehabilitation of the patients—in the establishment of these institutions social protection may be used as well as health protection; (b) specialized institutions for care and treatment of mental patients and sentenced criminal delinquents, for which the Secretariat for Internal Affairs (S.I.A.) and the Law Court services may be used, besides health protection; (c) specialized institutions for care and rehabilitation of children prevented from psychophysical development would play a very important role in enabling such children to achieve a more normal social life and in that way decrease the number of persons needing lifelong social care. In the organization of such institutions social protection and social insurance could be used, in addition to health protection; (d) specialized institutions for sociopathic children and the young, especially for underage delinquents, who are beginning to represent an increasing social and economical problem in our country. In this rehabilitation program the Service for the Protection of Mental Health could take part. The S.I.A. and the Law Court could provide the primary means for the establishment of these institutions; (e) specialized institutions for the rehabilitation and preventive and custodial care of patients suffering from cerebrovascular diseases. The number of these cases is constantly increasing while the possibilities of their cure are minimal; besides health protection it should be required that social insurance be used for that purpose; (f) specialized institutions for the care and treatment of geriatric patients who are selected from among those patients with psychiatric disorders and for whom there are no possibilities for accommodation and cure, although they increase in number constantly. In the organization of such institutions social protection should be used in addition to health protection.

All these specialized institutions should search for regional location and close coordination with the work of the general stationary institution. However, all stationary institutions for the protection of mental health must be organized in such a way as to unite curative, rehabilitative, and preventive activities. Their organic linking with the network of outpatient institutions is therefore necessary.

It cannot be overemphasized that the full efficacy of this program is possible only insofar as modern medical apparatus is available.

2. It is necessary and indispensable to improve the system of out-hospital protection of mental health, which represents the basic orientation of modern psychiatric service and which is very compatible with the communal system of health protection in our country.

In out-hospital protection a special place is occupied by the dispensaries, as the centers of the preventive, curative, and rehabilitative protection of mental health in local regions. Besides, the dispensaries ensure those who need their aid a normal life in their own environment, and ensure the maximal effectiveness of the activity with the minimal material contribution.

Complete dispensaries with diversified services for different mental disorders should be established in all developed medical centers without delay. Apart from that, it would be advisable that in smaller health localities, according to potentialities, small dispensaries and medical-pedagogical consulting institutions be formed. In addition, the development of dispensaries within the stationary or psychiatric institutions is an indispensable need.

The varied network of dispensaries of the general type has inevitably elucidated the need for special dispensaries for the protection of special groups of mentally disordered persons, such as alcoholics, epileptics, cerebrovascular, and geriatric mental patients, and depressed individuals.

In the complex prevention of mental illness, an important place should be given to the social and health institutions such as "homes," admission centers, workshops, and colonies. These have been established for mental patients who are not completely cured, or for those whose rehabilitation demands special measures and long time-periods (for instance, under-aged or adult delinquents). Such institutions should be included by plan into the network of dispensary institutions within the communal and local health centers.

The mental hygiene institutions should be viewed as the separate organic parts of the stationary and out-hospital institutions for health and protection. The latter would coordinate and integrate all the work relating to prevention of mental disorders and the improvement of mental health within the former.

3. In the organization of institutions for the protection of mental health the problem of personnel occupies one of the central places. Because of that it is necessary to pay attention to the education of personnel at all levels, from that of attendant to general practitioner and specialist. Within the system of education the obligation of learning basic things from the field of the protection of mental health should be introduced, as should be an obligatory working span for neuropsychiatrists.

Specific attention should be given to the educative development of sufficient medical and specialized personnel necessary for the maintainance of the appropriate institutions by providing for continued training. Besides that, means and institutions should be provided for the education of staffs which take part in the interdisciplinary mental health field, such as the following: psychologists, social workers and sociologists, pedagogists, defectologists, physiotherapists and work therapists.

4. The overall protection of mental health under modern social conditions demands permanent self-managing organs which could ensure and organize their own successful realization. For that purpose it is necessary to form a commission or a department for the protection of mental health in the health centers within one or more communities. The most advisable plan would be to incorporate these bodies into some of the existing institutions for the protection of mental health. The coordination of the work of these committees within republics and federations would be performed by existing commissions within the institutions for mental protection, or by permanent bodies of this type which would be formed.

5. To carry on successfully the protection of mental health the need for the improvements of conditions for scientific and research work should be emphasized.

At present, the need for formulating norms and making a classification of disorders, i.e., research work from the field of psychiatric epidemiology, is an urgent one. The means of these very important and very extensive investigations could be provided from the existing funds for scientific work, as well as from the social-insurance funds. The latter would be a positive decision economically because it would direct the health protection funds toward the appropriate decrease of psychiatric morbidity, which would affect a corresponding decrease in the cost of treatment of mental patients.

6. The unsolved question of psychiatric legislation represents a particular problem in the field of mental health. Because of that it is necessary, in the field of legislation, to revise the existing outdated regulations with the goal of creating a more complex law which would entirely regulate the protection of mental patients in their legal, possessional, civil and social relations. At the same time, this law would define the duties of our citizens toward mental patients, which would translate our legislation into the humanistic principles. [12, 29]

It should be mentioned that these recommendations are already being realized, particularly in the parts of the country which are relatively underdeveloped in the psychiatric sphere; they are given example and aid from the developed parts of the country. We believe that a new report, made several years later would be far clearer than this one is.

Yugoslav psychiatrists are optimistic about the future. They feel that they are able to realize the wish of their predecessors by their own efforts, that they can bring their work to a level on a par with that of world humanistic science. They are oriented to that by the progressive development of humanistic trends in all mankind and particularly by the predomination of these trends in their own environment.

References

1. M. BLEULER ET AL.: L'Enseignement de la psychiatrie et de l'hygiene mental; OMS, Geneva, 1962.
2. The Constitution of S.F.R.Y., Federal People's Assembly, Belgrade, 1963.
3. G. M. CROCETTI, A. KULCAR, B. KESIC, P. LEMKAU: Different Rates of Schizophrenia in Croatia, Yugoslavia, *American Journal of Public Health,* 54 (1964).
4. "Demographic Yearbook," United Nations, New York, 1961.
5. T. DJORDJEVIC: The Cure of Mentally Diseased in Monasteries, *The Herald of the Serbian Society of Science,* 3 (1928).
6. "Estimate of Working Ability of Socially Insured Persons Suffering from Neuropsychiatric Illnesses," Federal Institute for Social Insurance, Belgrade, 1964, 1965.
7. "General Law on Health Protection and Health Service," Narodno Zdravlje edition, Belgrade, 1965.
8. L. GLESINGER: The Foundation of the First Mental Hospitals in Croatia of the Twelfth Scientific Meeting of the Society for History of Medicine, Belgrade, 1964.
9. B. GOSTL: The History of Mental Hospital in Vrapce, *Neuropsychiatry,* (2) (1954).
10. The History of Medicine in Yugoslavia in "Medical Encyclopedia," vol. 8, Lexicographic Institute, Zagreb, 1963.
11. A. ILIC: The Role and Place of the Psychiatric Hospital in Belgrade in a Hundred Years Development of the Psychiatric Service in Serbia: *Serbian Archives for General Practice* (11) (1962).
12. "Information on the Situation and Problems in the Field of Mental Health Protection," Federal Commission for Mental Health, Belgrade, 1965.
13. "Instruction Plans and Programs of Faculties of Medicine in Belgrade, Zagreb, and Ljubljana."
14. "Instruction Plans and Programs of Faculties of Philosophy in Belgrade and Zagreb."
15. V. JAKOVLJEVIC: "Contr. a l'etude de l'influence psychologique des milieux culturels differents dans la pathogenie des neuroses," Clinique des maladies mentales, Paris, 1957.
16. ———: A Mental Health Center in an Underdeveloped Country (discussion); *International Journal of Psychiatry,* (2) (1965).
17. ———: "Milieu culturel et neuroses," *Ann. Med.-psych.,* Paris, 1962.
18. ———: La Survivance d'un rite culturel archaique—Fête des Roussales —sous forme de manifestations hysterique, Actes du VI Congr. int. des Sci. Anthr. et Ethnol., Paris, 1960.
19. ———: Transcultural-psychiatric Experiences from African Guinea; *Transc.-Psych. Rev.* 1 (1964).
20. D. JULIUS: "The Present State and Tasks of Neuro-Psychiatric Serv-

ice in FPRY," Papers Read at the Third Scientific Meeting of the Neuropsychiatrists, Medical Book, Belgrade, Zagreb, 1949.

21. M. KILIBARDA: "Development of Mental Disorders and Problems of Mental Health in the S.F.R.Y." Federal Institute for Health Protection, Belgrade, 1964.

22. ———: "Organization of Mental Health Protection in S.R.F.Y." *Narodno Zdravlje* (5) (1965).

23. P. LEMKAU AND A. PAVKOVIC: On the State of Psychiatric Health Service in Yugoslavia; in "The Problems and Tasks of Mental Hygiene," The Preventive of Health, Zagreb, 1952.

24. R. LOPASIC, S. BETLHEIM, AND S. DOGAN: "Psychiatry," Medical Book, Belgrade-Zagreb, 1959.

25. "Manual of the Intern. Statist. Classification of Diseases, Injuries and Causes of Death," WHO, Geneva, 1955.

26. Medicine in "Encyclopedia of Yugoslavia," vol. 6, Lexicographic Institute, Zagreb, 1965.

27. V. MILIC: Suicide in Yugoslavia, *Ann. of the Faculty of Law,* Belgrade, (3 and 4) (1959).

28. P. MILOSAVLJEVIC: The Foundation of the Mental Hospital in Belgrade and Its First Doctors; *Serbian Archives for General Practice,* (11) (1962).

29. "Minutes of Sessions of the Federal Commission For Mental Health," Federal Institute for Health Protection, Belgrade, 1964, 1965.

30. *Neuropsychiatry,* 2–10 (1953–1963); *Medical Courier* (special issues devoted to mental health) 1954 (11 and 12): 1961 (2 and 2a); 1964 (12).

31. N. PERSIC AND P. KOPORCIC: "Psychiatry and Neurology in the Service of the Preventive of Health," The Association of Health Institutions SR of Croatia, Zagreb, 1963.

32. "Programs of the First, Second, Third and Fourth Convention and the First and Second Congress of Yugoslav Neuropsychiatrists (1946, 1949, 1952, 1956, 1960, and 1964); Papers read at the Second Convention," Medicinska Knjiga edition, Belgrade, Zagreb, 1951; "Symposium on Neurosis," Third Congress of Serbian Doctors, The Serbian Medical Association, Belgrade, 1959; "Seminar on Mental Hygiene," Belgrade, 1960; "Symposium on Alcoholism," Zagreb, 1964.

33. "Regulations on Preparatory Service and Vocational Examinations, Terms of Specialized Studies and Specialist Examinations, Vocational Courses for Qualifying and Advanced Vocational Training of Employees of Health Institutions," Federal Secretariat for Public Health, Belgrade, 1948.

34. "Statistic Annual of the S.F.R.Y.," Federal Office of Statistics, Belgrade, 1950–1964.

35. V. STANOJEVIC: "The History of Medicine," Medical Book, Belgrade-Zagreb, 1953.

36. TSUNG-YI LIN AND C. C. STANDLEY: "La place de l'epidemiologie en psychiatrie," CMS, Geneva, 1963.

37. T. P. VUKANOVIC: Traitement des alienes dans les monasters chez les Slaves du Sud, L'Enthnographie (52) (1957).

38. "The Yearbook on Public Health and Health Service," Federal Institute for Health Protection, Belgrade, 1950–1964.

39. Yugoslavia, in "Encyclopedia of Yugoslavia," vol. 5, Lexicographic Institute, Zagreb, 1960.

CHAPTER SIX

Czechoslovak Psychiatry

BY
DR. JOSEF PROKUPEK, DR. JAROSLAV STUCHLIK
AND DR. STANISLAV GROF

HISTORICAL SURVEY

THE CZECHOSLOVAK SOCIALIST REPUBLIC is a continental middle European state with a territory of 127,859 square kilometers and a population of fourteen million. Historically it is composed of three countries: Bohemia, Moravia-Silesia, and Slovakia. The first two countries are inhabited by people of Czech nationality (approximately 66 percent of the total population); in Slovakia another ethnic group prevails—the Slovaks, who comprise approximately 28 percent of the whole population. The remaining 5 percent consists of Hungarians, Ukrainians, and Germans.

The first care of psychotic patients in Bohemia dates back to the tenth century. At that time, so-called "spitals" in monasteries provided shelter and asylum for the mentally ill.

The foundation of Prague University—the first university in middle Europe—by the emperor Charles IV in 1348 contributed to the elevation of the cultural level in Bohemia and to the development of medicine.

In 1458 the first autonomous asylum for psychotics was established in Znojmo, Moravia. In 1783 an asylum for the mentally ill was founded by the clergy in Prague at the Hospital of Misericordial Brethren.

In 1790 the first special facilities for the mentally ill with 57 one-bed rooms were established in Prague within the bounds of the general hospital. Later developments weakened this connection of psychiatry with somatic medicine, and new institutes for psychiatric patients were arranged independently, usually at a considerable distance from big towns and public hospitals.

Jan Theobald Held lectured on psychiatry to students of medicine and accompanied his lectures with demonstrations of patients. He advocated a materialistic basis for the psychoses and in 1812 wrote: "Thinking is a certain kind of chemical process."

He recommended that pathological psychic activity be studied by means of physics and physiology. Held correctly pointed to the importance of environmental factors with regard to the origin and development of mental diseases: in 1811 he connected the higher occurrences of psychic disturbances with the deterioration of social conditions after the state bankruptcy; and he refused the idealistic explanation that the increase in the number of the ill was caused by the fact that a new comet had appeared in the sky at that time. Held also directed the new Prague psychiatric hospital of St. Catherine, which was adapted from a former monastery. In 1829 this institute had 260 beds, and later the number was increased to 500.

Under the Austro-Hungarian monarchy giant institutes were set up in Prague-Bohnice and Kromeriz, Moravia, both of which were large enough to hold more than 2,000 patients. The older establishments, such as those at Dobrany and Berkovice, Bohemia, and at Brno and Sternberg, Moravia, answered fully the purpose of detention. Occupational therapy was systematically applied on institute-owned landed estates.

The setting up of open departments not requiring legal formalities for detention was not put in action until after 1918, first in Slovakia at Nitra, Levare, Trencin, and Levoca, and later in Bohemia.

The main contributor in the period from 1787 to 1869 was Jan Evangelista Purkyne. His work in the field of psychology of senses is well known. He contributed to the development of psychiatry through his studies on the morphology of cells and physiological studies on the action of organs as well as through the development of methodology and experimental physiology.

A school of positivistic psychology grew under Wundt and Spencer's

influences. The founder and leader of this orientation was Frantisek
Krejci (1858–1934), professor of psychology at the University of Prague.
In the five volumes of his comprehensive *Textbook of Psychology*, 1902–
1909, a good deal of psychical pathology was described which influenced
the positivistic thinking of some psychiatrists.

Other philosophical schools, such as those of materialism and
Thomism, also flourished in this period.

In 1844 the "New House" was built in the garden of the Prague
Hospital. At that time it was the most modern psychiatric facility in
Europe. Psychiatrists from all over the world came to see the equipment
and the methods of work. Besides pharmacotherapy (mainly sedative),
rehabilitation was advanced by physical therapy (hydrotherapy and the
drinking of mineral waters from Karlsbad), occupational therapy, physical
training, and musicotherapy. These progressive methods were introduced
by J. B. Riedl, who in 1840 became the first reader in psychiatry. His
follower F. Kostel later introduced the inoculation of artificial variola in
patients with general paresis and thus became the inventor of therapy by
means of artificially evoked high temperatures.

When the University of Prague was divided into a Czech part
(Charles University) and a German part, Professor K. Kuffner, the
founder of modern Czech psychiatry, became the head of the Charles
University Department of Psychiatry. He was an adherent of the materialistic conception of psychiatry (as was his contemporary German colleague W. Griesinger). He saw the causes of psychic disturbances in
the defective development of the central nervous system and in diseases
of the brain. He pointed out that mental disturbances have regular pathological causes and a characteristic development and course (in a similar way
to that which E. Kraepelin later formulated with respect to his nosological
entities). Kuffner presupposed in the cases of mental diseases in which no
pathologically anatomical lesion of the central nervous system was de-
tectable a "disturbance of production, discharge and displacement of energy
in psychic centers and tracts."

The first *Textbook of Psychiatry*, by Karel Kuffner (1858–1939),
was published in 1897. It laid the foundations for the Czech scientific
psychiatric terminology. It was organistic in its nosological conception and
descriptive in its psychological parts. Most published works in psychiatry
from the latter half of the nineteenth century to World War I consisted
predominantly of casuistic studies. Symptomatological minuteness, comprehensive clinical description, a tendency toward accurate pathological

anatomical findings and relations, and phenomenological systemization were characteristic of these works, as was a lack of philosophical or noetic aspects and basic conceptions.

It can be viewed as typical of this trend that Kuffner's disciple Jan Jansky (1873–1929), professor of psychiatry at the University of Prague, became well known for his independent discovery of blood groups before Landsteiner. Another of Kuffner's disciples, Leo Taussig (1884–1944), professor of psychiatry at the University of Prague, became prominent for his works in liquorology, or the study of cerebrospinal fluid.

The immediate successor to Kuffner for the Prague psychiatric chair, Professor Zdenek Myslivecek, published a number of studies on the spinal cord and brain histology, some contributions to the histology of syringomyelia and sclerosis amyotrophica, and some descriptive psychological articles treating of symptomological syndromes. In 1949 he published a *Textbook of General Psychiatry.*

The psychiatric department of the School of Medicine at Prague was the only university institution in the state until the end of World War I. This situation led undoubtedly to one advantage: All physicians had a uniform education in psychiatry. In this way materialistic conceptions of Kuffner became deeply rooted and no extravagant doctrines were accepted, as was the case from time to time in foreign psychiatry. Immediate foreign sources that influenced our psychiatrists can be found in German, Austrian, French, and Russian psychiatry, but the influences were more in theory than in practice.

A more profound conception of psychiatry was introduced by Antonin Heveroch. His textbook on *The Diagnostics of Mental Disease* (1904) followed the pattern of Kraepelin's Einfuhrung. It dealt with casuistry as well as analysis and systematic considerations and considered general and special therapy, forensic consequences, and even social inferences. In the field of research he distinguished himself by his comprehensive and profound examination of the problem of aphasias. In the field of psychology he became absorbed in the problem of the self, or selfhood, which, however, came to be classed by French psychiatrists among the depersonalization disorders in general and to be understood as a schizophrenic split by Bleuler.

At least fifty years ago, the problem of consciousness came to be the central problem that Czech philosophers, psychologists, and psychiatrists dealt with. Among the physicians, Ladislav Haskovec (1866–1944) urged the view that the seat of consciousness was in the area surrounding the third and fourth ventricles of the brain. Heveroch's pupil Otakar Janota gave special attention to the problems of depersonalization as well as to the psychological side of the study of psychoses. Another pupil of Heveroch's, Vladimir Vondracek, devoted a number of studies to the several sectors of psychology in general. His monograph *"On Perception"* is written from the standpoint of physiological psychology. Having studied pharmacology as well, he discussed it in his book *Pharmacology of the Mind* (1935). He also made several concrete contributions to the psychology of the treatment of psychical disorders.

The psychological trend in psychiatry is represented by Jaroslav Stuchlik, Professor Emeritus of Psychiatry, University of Bratislava, formerly head of the Psychiatric University Clinic in Pilsen. From Kraepelin, with whom he had studied, he acquired a tendency toward minute symptomatological psychological analysis; and from Bleuler, in whose clinic he was active, an inclination toward an analytical mastering of the doctrines of depth psychologies and a critical attitude toward psychoanalysis; and from Freud, to whose Vienna circle he belonged, the determination to master the psychology of depth states. He devoted himself to experimental psychology, to the elaboration of nosological psychiatric entities, especially the notion of psychosis in general, to the study and application of all forms of psychotherapy from hypnosis to persuasion, to forensic psychiatry, and to the problem of epilepsy.

He advanced definitions of the new nosological units: the pathophronesias and the habit states. Pathophronesia is an all-embracing concept of the deformed connection between the somatic basis of a given state and the psychic or somatic corresponding manifestations. Hypophronesia, "undersensibility," is a disturbance of intelligence characterized by a certain poorness of associative activity and an incapability of the subject's own judgment about contents and values of thought. Habit states are conceived of as various syndromes which persist after their organic or functional origin has ceased to exist.

Dr. Stuchlik was the first to introduce psychoanalysis in Czech literature and practice. The Psychoanalytical Society of Czechoslovakia was established by Emanuel Windholz and was later conducted by Bohodar Dosuzkov.

After World War I two new universities were established in Brno and Bratislava. After World War II additional universities were founded in Hradec Kralove, Pilsen, Olomouc, and Kosice. In this way needed conditions were created not only for the education of a necessary number of new physicians but also for scientific work which was carried out in the psychiatric departments of these schools of medicine.

Psychiatric hospitals, formerly called country lunatic asylums, were for the past century established in either old monasteries or castles not always satisfactorily adapted or were formerly special functional buildings that had served their purpose until the present. The network of mental hospitals in the Czech countries was adequate. However, in Slovakia, which was neglected so far as sanitary service is concerned, there was a considerable lack of psychiatric beds, alleviated only by psychiatric departments of great hospitals. (This situation had the advantage already mentioned of sustaining a closer cooperation with other medical branches.) The lack could not be fully dealt with until the present.

After the year 1953, psychiatric departments in hospitals (besides those in Slovakia) were established in greater number. These departments significantly contributed to the fact that prejudices against psychiatry among the nonmedical population gradually disappeared. Mental hospitals, because of previous little therapeutic activity, had been thought of formerly as the "last resort" of the patient. As long as the care for psychotics was predominantly limited to keeping them in an asylum, there was no need for a greater number of paramedical personnel with higher qualifications. The development of therapy in psychiatry, especially during the past fifteen years, and the use of forms of psychiatric care evoked the need for a greater number of qualified personnel and for new equipment (day rooms, laboratories, etc.). Thus the interest in psychiatry increased even among students of medicine, and it has lasted, whether or not the students have specialized in psychiatry or in other medical disciplines. The development of psychosomatic medicine has helped to maintain this trend.

The mental hygiene movement was introduced into our country by Jaroslav Stuchlik in 1921 on the initiative of the Ligue D'Hygiene Mentale of Paris. It developed under the guidance of the Czechoslovak Society for Mental Health and with substantial state subsidies. One of the foremost representatives of this movement, Matej Brandejs (1869–1941), head of the Prague asylum, edited the renowned periodical *The Mind* and represented Czechoslovakia in the first international congresses of mental hygiene in Washington, D.C., and Paris. This movement has continued its work under the guidance of Jaroslav Stuchlik, assisted by Secretary-General Jiri Semotan and in cooperation with quite a number of psychiatrists and other specialists.

During World War II and for almost ten years after its termination,

Czechoslovak psychiatry was isolated from the world of psychiatry. This has changed in recent years with a richer exchange of personal visits and publications between countries. Czech psychiatry still basically maintains the materialistic conception, which ensures that it shall retain its scientific foundations and will not slip into doubtful theories and practices that only formally resemble the scientific approach. Fifteen years ago our psychiatry had an occasion to become more deeply oriented to the neurophysiological doctrine of I. P. Pavlov. Now it critically evaluates this doctrine, as well as all other doctrines and methods used in the world and tries to accept their more vital cores. The Pavlovian doctrine supplied not only the reflex principle of psychic activities but also the concepts of the formative influence of outer environment, the integrity of the individual, and the milieu. This has played an important role in the problems of the etiopathogenesis of psychic disturbances as well as in the introduction of new forms of psychiatric care and new principles of mental health care to the whole population. Mental health care, which we used to call mental hygiene, has become a foremost task for psychiatry because of its immense social significance, and it is a realization of the program of our physiologist J. E. Purkyne, who wrote in the year 1823:

The task of the physician is not only to restore life and prolong it for a short time, but to protect it from corruption and help it to attain the summit of admirable perfection and beauty.
Attention is not yet paid to the fact that medicine will not be perfect in all its aspects until—as far as this is at all possible in face of such great changeability and hostility of external forces—it starts teaching how to invigorate the fragile human organism, how to prevent affection and combat illness, and until it is capable of performing these tasks in such a way as to enable human life that was well conceived to pass through all its phases, properly adapting itself both to the limits of the individual and of the society, and to be happily and gloriously perfected to its natural end.

This vision of Purkyne's, valid also in psychiatry and mental health care, was brought forth at the time of the suppression of the Czech nation during the capitalist era, but it can also become a reality in the contemporaneous conditions of our socialist society. The document of the party and of the government about the care for health from the year 1964 not only stresses the claims that the citizens have with respect to health but it also gives them a duty to care for their health and to create healthy living conditions. It also stresses the importance of factors of psychological character on health; and it gives orders to maintain the principles of mental hygiene.

PSYCHIATRIC CARE IN CZECHOSLOVAKIA TODAY

While the development of psychiatry after World War II did not proceed as rapidly as other medical disciplines, it benefited from them. The development of venerologic service led to a substantial decrease in the occurence of general paresis. Similarly, the number of postpartum psychoses was considerably reduced, because nearly all the deliveries in the Czechoslovak Socialist Republic were carried out in expert institutes under aseptic conditions.

The foundations for the postwar development of psychiatry were laid in 1953, when a group of progressive psychiatrists elaborated the program of psychiatric care. New tasks for psychiatry were stated: better outpatient psychiatric care and prevention of mental diseases with continuous development and improvement of inpatient facilities; the necessity for training new physicians and paramedical personnel; the establishment of psychiatric service for children; more efficient forms of fighting alcoholism and improvements of its treatment; exploration of new methods of therapy, rehabilitation, and resocialization for psychiatric patients, etc.

Gradually, improved therapeutic results contributed highly to the fact that psychiatry, which heretofore had not had the same authority as other medical disciplines, began to reach an equivalent position among them.

In 1958, the Ministry of Health included for the first time psychiatry among its chief tasks. By this act, the necessary organizational basis was formed for removing numerous deficiencies in the care of the mentally ill.

The basic principles of the Czechoslovak care can be summarized as follows: Theoretical foundations are materialistic, based on reflex theory. They influence the organizational forms of psychiatric care. In diagnostic, clinical, therapeutic, and rehabilitation practice, Czechoslovak psychiatry makes use of all modern scientific methods. It requires not only high qualifications for psychiatric personnel but also good apparatuses and other equipment. Emphasis is on outpatient services (day and night hospitals and sheltered workshops included), which are expected to facilitate adequate prophylaxis and the systematic introduction of follow-up care. Child psychiatry and the fight against alcoholism are an inseparable part of the psychiatric program. Clinical observation is the basis of the psychiatric examination; however, it makes use of the results of biochemical, neurophysical, psychological, sociological, and other laboratory methods.

The Psychiatric Research Institute has the right and duty to lead method-ologically the research in psychiatry that is carried out in all the work-ing places throughout the republic. Psychiatric care is carried out accord-ing to the plan of development of the sanitary services with a certain pref-erence for and agreement with the economical development. To be able to offer the best medical and sanitary help all physicians and the paramedi-cal personnel are obliged to improve their qualifications by further train-ing. Central control of psychiatric help enables it to reach a uniform and high level in all parts of the state.

Psychiatric care is a part of the state medical care and is governed by the Ministry of Public Health. The majority of the mental health serv-ices and programs for the mentally ill and handicapped are administered by the Department for Therapeutic and Preventive Care, which has an administrator-psychiatrist on the staff. Scientific consultation and expert control of the mental health services are entrusted to the chief psychiatrist of the Ministry of Health. He cooperates with the advisory committee of psychiatrists, composed of a number of leading psychiatrists from the whole country.

At the regional level, mental health services are administered by the regional national committees through their health departments, headed by a physician. The regional psychiatrist is an expert psychiatrist, who is assisted by a regional advisory committee of psychiatrists.

At the district level, mental health services are controlled by the district national committees with their health departments. Medical direc-tors of local inpatient and outpatient facilities also participate in the administration of mental health services in individual districts.

PSYCHIATRIC INPATIENT CARE

The main task of psychiatric care was always inpatient care, which was evolved earlier than other forms. The tradition of inpatient psychiatric care created rigid stereotypes, which were often difficult obstacles to efforts to introduce new principles of treatment in psychiatric hospitals. A more advantageous situation exists in newly established psychiatric departments in hospitals, the activity of which can be more progressive. The hospitalization of psychiatric patients is also carried out in some sanatariums in spas; and a smaller number of patients are treated also in the somatic departments of general hospitals (especially neurotics), in facilities for social care of invalids, and in homes for elderly persons. To obtain the needed number of beds for psychiatric patients (psychically ill and mentally defective), some beds in special childrens' institutions and other facilities of educative and rehabilitory care must be added.

Mental Hospitals

The network of mental hospitals is not displaced with regard to the density of the population. Therefore territories which refer to particular hospitals are exactly determined, and in the majority of such cases they coincide with the districts of the pertinent regions where they are situated.

In the year 1937, there were 16,909 beds in mental hospitals in the Czechoslovak Republic, which represented more than 23 percent of all hospital beds. After World War II, a reduction in the number of beds occurred, because mental hospitals were not further developed. (After World War I a similar decrease of hospitalized psychotics was noted.) The deficit reached its maximum in the year 1949 when there was a reduction of more than one-third in comparison with the prewar situation. In the meantime, a rapid increase of the number of the beds in hospitals occurred in connection with the fact that all sanitary care including hospitalization was free of charge and therefore increasing use was made of them. Before World War II only persons paying the medical-insurance fees could claim hospitalization free of charge, and then only for a limited period (twenty-eight to sixty days in a year). Accordingly psychiatric beds represented only approximately twelve percent of the total capacity of hospital beds, i.e., 0.91 psychiatric beds to 1,000 inhabitants in comparison with the previous ratio of 1.17 to 1,000.

In 1957 the prewar level was reached with regard to psychiatric beds, if beds in psychiatric departments of general hospitals were included: thirteen percent of the total number of hospital beds were psychiatric, and there was a ratio of 1.27 psychiatric beds to 1,000 inhabitants.

Toward the end of 1963 there were 16,546 beds in psychiatric hospitals in the Czechoslovak Socialist Republic. (To this, in addition, 2,137 beds in psychiatric services of general hospitals must be added, which represents a total of 18,683 beds, 10.9 percent of all hospital beds and a ratio of 1.36 to 1,000 inhabitants.)

Psychiatric hospitals not only serve for treating acute cases of psychic diseases, but also are suited for long-term hospitalization. The time of treatment in psychiatric hospitals shortened gradually as a result of the complex approach and use of modern methods of therapy. In 1955, the average duration of hospitalization was 262 days; in 1962, only 190 days.

The exploitation of the capacity of beds exceeded 100 percent in some mental hospitals; on the average it amounted to 98.8 percent in 1959. At the end of 1960 this rate decreased substantially; and in 1962 it amounted to only 92 percent.

The rotation of patients on the beds increased; the number of readmitted patients increased at the same time from 33 percent in 1958 to 50.3 percent in 1963.

Until 1959 the number of admitted patients was higher than that of the discharged ones, so a systematic overcrowding of mental hospitals resulted. Since then discharged patients have outnumbered admitted patients.

The enhanced activity of psychiatric hospitals was made possible mainly by the fact that the number of doctors increased substantially. In 1949 there was 1 physician to 160 beds, whereas in 1963 only 1 to 53.6 beds. Also, the nurses participated more in expert activities. This was made possible by the fact that 80 percent of the paramedical personnel had full qualifications and that expert professions of rehabilitation staff were established. The lack of interest of men in nursing activity (for which they are paid less than in work in industrial enterprises) was partly solved by employing female nurses even in departments for male patients. Also the participation of psychologists in the diagnostic and therapeutic process under the control of physicians contributed highly to the increase of the quality and efficiency of the treatment.

In some large general hospitals mixed neurological-psychiatric wards were established. When in the Czechoslovak Socialist Republic neurology was separated from psychiatry (in 1955), there was a great development of special psychiatric services, especially in regional hospitals, but also in some district hospitals. In the cities, where the regional hospital is a part of the school of medicine of the university, the psychiatric department is at the same time a pedagogic facility.

The psychiatric services of general hospitals soon acquired a good reputation among the general population and the surviving prejudices against psychiatry were not connected with them as was the case with psychiatric hospitals. Although their capacity formed approximately 11 percent of the total number of psychiatric beds, they handled about thirty-nine percent of all psychiatric hospitalizations. The structure of diagnostic groups did not at the same time substantially differ from that in psychiatric hospitals (only fewer senile and atherosclerotic psychoses were admitted). Also the length of hospitalization in the psychiatric departments of general hospitals was incomparably shorter—forty-three days, approximately. Some of the admitted patients came only for the sake of observation or to form a judgment about their health condition. A greater rotation of patients was made possible by the fact that the psychiatric services of general hospitals were granted more medical personnel—there was a ratio of 1 physician to 22–24 patients. The advantages of the psychiatric services of general hospitals are severalfold. Psychiatric care is closer to the population: Psychiatric departments are now in larger towns, unlike the mental hospitals. There is more cooperation with other departments of the hospitals and it is possible readily to use consulting services for hospitalized patients and also to offer psychiatric consulting service to patients in somatic departments. Incipient psychotic conditions can be admitted and subdued with early treatment (whereas many physicians as well as patients and their relatives hesitate in the case of hospitalization in a mental hospital). Admission to the psychiatric service of a general hospital is handled in the same way as it is in other departments of the hospitals, i.e., without restrictions by legal regulations of an administrative character. These departments contribute to more correct views of psychic disturbances in the lay population.

Psychiatric services of general hospitals are mostly on a small capacity and are not suited for long-term patients. There is not as much opportunity for an all-out rehabilitation of the mentally ill. Therefore, they cooperate closely with the appropriate mental hospitals and form with them (and with the outpatient psychiatric care) a functional unit administratively.

The experiences acquired are an incentive for establishing more departments of this kind in general hospitals rather than additional mental hospitals.

Czechoslovakia is rich in spas with mineral waters and favorable climatic conditions—some of them are world famous (Karlsbad, Marienbad, Piešťany, Jeseník). In many spas, not only neurotics but also persons who have undergone a psychotic episode can improve their health, especially in Jeseník (formerly Grafenberg) which has an old tradition in this respect. Treatment in spas is free for working people, but it must be prescribed by a psychiatrist. In the last few years in six spas conditions were created for expert treatment and rehabilitation of psychotic patients. The bed capacity of these places is about 600 beds in total.

Outpatient Care

The development of outpatient mental health care in the Czechoslovak Socialist Republic did not begin until after World War II, in agreement with the general conception of health service with stress upon preventive care. A lack of specialized physicians was the reason that development could not progress at a necessary speed. It was indispensable to educate doctors for responsible outpatient work. Therefore, at the beginning, physicians from inpatient psychiatric facilities participated in outpatient service on a part-time basis. Some psychiatrists could become fully dedicated to outpatient service and at the same time (usually once in a week) work at inpatient clinics where their patients were hospitalized.

Whereas in the first years there was little interest among organizers of medical care in the functioning of the psychiatric outpatient services in the district, the situation has changed now to such an extent that it is not even possible to cover their requirements.

In outpatient psychiatric service we now see the main task as psychiatric care and therefore we give preference to it. According to the plan, the ratio of 0.25 psychiatrists to 10,000 inhabitants should be reached in the whole territory of the state. This means that in districts which have about 100,000 inhabitants 2.5 psychiatrists shall practice. This will make possible team work and specialization for certain components of psychiatric care (child psychiatry, anti-alcoholic fight, etc.). It will also make possible dispensary services and active searches for persons threatened by mental disorder as well as therapeutic and rehabilitation care for patients in their familial and professional milieu.

The number of appointments per hour amounts to 2.5 patients. In 1963, 597,837 appointments were carried out in psychiatric outpatient services and 197,252 persons were examined for the first time, i.e., nearly 32 percent of all appointments. For persons examined for the first time, the following percentages of diagnoses were made: psychosis, 21 percent; neurosis, 43 percent; alcoholism, 10 percent; psychopathy, 13 percent.

The tasks of the ambulatory psychiatric service can be summarized as follows:

1. Make the diagnosis of the psychic disorder and of the therapeutic and rehabilitation plan (in the future it is planned that the local

and family doctors will treat their patients according to the advice of the psychiatrist; their education is directed toward this)

2. Look for evidence of morbidity with mental disorders or of persons endangered by them
3. Make an active search for persons with mental disorders or for persons endangered by them
4. Create social, sanitary, and preventive care
5. Provide a consulting service for other medical disciplines
6. Give sanitary education to the population
7. Include research and teaching in selected working places.

We do not see the psychiatric outpatient care as an emergency facility, which should reduce the claims for hospitalization by patients, but we see a new quality of psychiatric care in it.

Psychiatric care for children is ensured in the outpatient service by experts always for two (or more) neighboring districts. Anti-alcoholic outpatient care is ensured by antialcoholic consulting centers that are in all districts attached to the psychiatric outpatient services. Their activity is supplemented by the emergency centers for persons intoxicated by alcohol. These stations work in the larger cities. In 1963, there were forty such stations with 356 beds.

Day Hospitals and Night Hospitals

Day and night hospitals represent a supplement of the outpatient psychiatric service and a transitional facility to inpatient care. They afforded good service abroad, because they provided contact for the patient with his familial or professional milieu. At present the Ministry of Health has issued directives for establishing them. In recent years, this system was used in several inpatient facilities for some patients, who lived in their environment. Experiences gained were valuable and they showed that in this way it is possible to shorten the time of treatment and accelerate the process of resocialization after active therapy.

The contact of hospitalized patients with their families is much more extensive than it was before, and the patients can visit their homes. Even this arrangement, as well as the open-door policy introduced in inpatient facilities, helps provide a more rapid improvement of the morbid condition.

PSYCHIATRIC PERSONNEL AND THEIR TRAINING

The job of offering good psychiatric care and evolving care for mental health cannot be fulfilled without qualified personnel and without systematically heightening their standards.

Education in psychiatry is realized in relatively few lessons in the schools of medicine—only three hours of letcures and three hours of practical training a week during a single semester. It is therefore necessary that the newly graduated doctors who begin to practice in psychiatry extend their basic knowledge gradually during their clinical work. The Psychiatric Department of the Postgraduate Medical Training Institute, established in 1955, has prepared a model plan of individual study for them, covering a period of three years, after which they must pass an attestation examination before a state commission. Young doctors work under the supervision of expert psychiatrists who should also test the results of their private study. They also participate actively in expert work at staff conferences in their hospital and at conferences organized by the psychiatric section of the Czechoslovak Medical Association under J. E. Purkyně. To facilitate the preparation of young physicians for the specialization attestation examination, the psychiatric department of the Postgraduate Medical Training Institute holds special courses for doctors before attestation that last three months. In these ways, they can supplement their expert theoretical and practical knowledge, especially in areas in which they had not the occasion to learn in their working place. The specialization attestation has a theoretical and a practical part, which consists of a complete examination of a patient that includes determining the diagnosis, differentially diagnostic considerations, further investigation treatment program, etc.

For psychiatric specialists the psychiatric departments of the Postgraduate Medical Training Institute (in Prague and Bratislava) have organized postgraduate courses which are cyclic and run in intervals of three years. These are directed either to the functional position of the physicians (for chief doctors, psychiatrists in outpatient service, etc.) or to certain themes (forensic expertise, psychotherapy, etc.). All courses are free of charge and the doctors get their full incomes for this time.

In addition, for separate sectors of mental health care, special training posts are arranged that enable the doctors to learn more fully pertinent problems (e.g., EEG, examination of cerebrospinal fluid, child psychiatry, etc.) in theory as well as practice.

Besides the doctors, other specialists with university education work in psychiatric facilities—for example, psychologists, biochemists, etc. Their number has gradually increased with increasing needs for experts.

Paramedical personnel have become more and more significant co-workers of the doctors. Their training lasts four years, and it is received in sanitary schools, from which come qualified nurses, laboratory assistants, rehabilitation assistants, etc. Also, the number of social nurses has increased with the extension of care for the ill and the increased socially legal support. A minority (about 20 percent) of paramedical personnel is composed of auxiliary nurses and unqualified sanitary personnel. On the average, there is 1 paramedical employee to 5.7 patients in a mental hospital. Similarly, as do the doctors so also do the paramedical employees get during their employment systematic additional education in the form of lessons or participation in programs prepared by the Institute for Further Training of Paramedical Personnel. The incomes of workers in psychiatry are better because of a special allowance in other disciplines in comparison with workers and also their holidays are a week longer.

PSYCHIATRIC RESEARCH

Psychiatric research in Czechoslovakia is governed and controlled by the Ministry of Public Health. The organizational and methodological center of psychiatric research is the Psychiatric Research Institute in Prague, which is directly subordinated to the Ministry of Public Health.

Two psychiatric problems are included in the *state plan of research* as serious diseases endangering the health of people. One is prevention and therapy of neuroses, which includes study of social and biological conditions that contribute to the development of neurotic disorders, experimental study of maladaptive manifestations and reactions, and comparative study of the therapy of neuroses. The other is psychopathies: pathogenesis, diagnosis, and therapy.

Furthermore, there are several thematic areas of research that belong to the *resort plan;* their importance is considered to be more or less limited to psychiatry as a scientific discipline. The *research on biological factors in schizophrenia* includes the study of somatic and neurophysiological manifestations of this disease, especially of biochemical, immunochemical, electroencephalographic and motor changes, and changes of higher nervous activity.

The *research in the area of emotional disorders* and emotional factors in etiopathogenesis, therapy, and prevention of psychic and corticovisceral disease comprises studies concerning the mechanism of emotional disorders from the psychopathological, physiological, pathophysiological, biochemical, and sociological points of view.

The *research in genetic factors in psychic disorders* deals with epidemiological, clinical, and humoral studies of genetic factors in connection with basic genetic research.

The *research in psychiatric epidemiology* concerns study of general psychiatric morbidity by means of epidemiological and statistical methods with special regard to depressive conditions, suicidal rate, readmissions of psychiatric patients, infantile morbidity, etc.

The *research in the field of rehabilitation in psychiatry* includes study of the hospital milieu and its influence on the treatment and course of psychoses, of the occupational therapy, and of psychiatric rehabilitation by means of clinical and psychological methods.

A very important part of research is the *study of psychotropic drugs,* which is included in the pharmacological resort plan. Here special attention is being given to an extensive comparative study of ataractic and antidepressive drugs which is being carried out in a standard way and under double-blind conditions in many psychiatric in and outpatient facilities. A study of this kind was made possible by the uniform organizational basis of the Czechoslovak health care. This research program was prepared and is being controlled by the psychopharmacological department of the Psychiatric Research Institute in Prague.

Each of the above thematic areas mentioned of the state and resort plan of research has a chief organizer and central working place. The research of specific problems in separate thematic areas is carried out by different individual workers or teams of workers in the Psychiatric Research Institute, medical faculties, postgraduate medical training centers, mental hospitals, outpatient service, and other psychiatric facilities. The chief organizer of the psychiatric research in the whole C.S.S.R. is the director of the Psychiatric Research Institute.

The Psychiatric Research Institute started functioning on January 1, 1961; up until now it has been the only psychiatric research institute in Czechoslovakia. It is headed by a director working with a scientific council composed of outstanding representatives from psychiatry and neighboring disciplines from all over the country. For internal purposes he has, in addition, a research council composed of only Institute members. The institute has four research units: for the study of psychopathies, neuroses, psychotropic drugs, and schizophrenia. The separate research topics are included in either the state or the resort plan of research of the Ministry of Health.

A great advantage for the research in Czechoslovakia is the uniform structure and organization of mental health service, which allows for close connection and cooperation between research and practice.

TREATMENT

The beginnings of modern psychiatric treatment can be traced back to 1936 when insulin and cardiazol were introduced into therapy; wider use of new therapeutic methods roughly coincides with the beginning of World War II. Convulsive methods of therapy, which appeared at this time, prevailed in psychiatry for many years following. In agreement with the practice in other countries, electroconvulsive treatment was widely used in manic-depressive disorders in the form of a series of singular shocks in the case of depressions or as a cumulative treatment in serious manic manifestations. Also several modifications of electroconvulsive therapy (electronarcosis, sliding electroconvulsions, and later electroshocks with pretreatment by muscle-relaxant drugs) were commonly used. In schizophrenic cases, electroconvulsive therapy was recommended for stationary clinical pictures with marked inhibition or catatonic stupor, whereas for acute forms and paranoid conditions insulin convulsive therapy was administered. As far as insulin is concerned, it was also used in subcomatous doses, mainly in less marked depressive disorders and involutional melancholy. Besides electric and insulin shock therapy, cardiazol and acetylcholine were also applied for evoking therapeutic convulsions; however, they were used to a much smaller extent than were the former ones. These forms of therapy were supplemented by the administration of hypnotics, vegetative regulatory drugs, hydrotherapy, and occupational therapy in various combinations. In some cases pyretotherapy, widely used in general paresis, was also applied in endogenous psychoses.

As far as psychosurgery is concerned, prefrontal lobotomy was performed in severe schizophrenic states and conditions of uncontrollable excitement and aggressivity, especially in stubborn obsessive-compulsive disorders. This approach never reached wide acceptance, however, and after 1952, it was completely abandoned in Czechoslovakia. The rough methods of these surgical interventions that were known at that time were believed to have little scientific foundation, were not sufficiently controllable, and caused devastating damage to the brain of the patients. In recent years, a renewed interest in psychosurgery can be observed in the form of precisely focused microsurgical interventions.

In 1955, two major ataractics, chlorpromazine and reserpine, were introduced in psychiatric therapy in Czechoslovakia, and this meant the beginning of a new era. Since that time, many major and minor tranquilizing drugs and recently also antidepressants have enriched the psychiatric therapeutic armamentarium. Czechoslovak psychiatrists have been able to work with the majority of psychotropic drugs of foreign origin and the pharmaceutical industry of the country produces those that have proved clinically most useful. The Research Institute for Pharmacy and Biochemistry, moreover, has synthetized several original Czechoslovak psychotropic drugs.Wide use of ataractic and antidepressive drugs has replaced to a great extent convulsive treatments, which have been reserved mostly only for those cases for which drugs have proved ineffectual. At present, both kinds of psychiatric therapy are widely used.

As was the case in other countries, the ataractic era effected a revolution in mental hospitals. Their basic character underwent a substantial change: nowadays patients with psychomotor excitation and aggressive manifestations cannot be found in the wards and beds with protective nets and isolation rooms are no longer necessary. Even the patients in psychotic wards have become more socialized, and the overall outlook of many wards does not basically differ from departments for somatic patients. Grilles have gradually disappeared from the windows of mental hospitals and open-door policies have been introduced in many pavilions.

As far as psychotherapy is concerned, it is generally acknowledged that it represents an important and indispensable method, which should accompany any other therapeutic approach. It is widely used in its unspecific forms (encouragement, support, persuasion, suggestion, reeducation, consulting, rational explanation, etc.). In several places in Czechoslovakia hypnosis and autogenous training is being systematically used for therapeutic purposes. Rational, dynamically oriented psychotherapy was not used on a broader scale until the last decade.

Psychoanalysis, even though historically it is closely linked to our country (Freud's birthplace was Príbor in Moravia), has never achieved a wide acceptance. A small society for the study of psychoanalysis in Prague working before World War II was weakened by the emigration of its members to the West, and during the Nazi occupation the rest of it functioned illegally. After the war, it existed only several years and was dissolved in 1950.*

The development of Czechoslovak's dynamic psychotherapy mentioned above can be characterized, in contradistinction to orthodox Freudian analysis, by an interpersonal orientation and a great regard to social factors. The first center of dynamic psychotherapy was established in the Faculty Policlinics in Prague, which is a part of the medical faculty of Charles University. Here the patients, mostly neurotics, attend regular group and collective psychotherapeutic sessions. A Czechoslovak specialty is the Rehabilitation Center for Neurotics, which is attached to the psychiatric department of Faculty Policlinics. It is situated sixty kilometers from Prague in a small castle and has thirty beds for both male and female patients. Here, ergotherapy is combined with a complex program of collective psychotherapy and psychogymnastics. Patients whose condition requires a special approach are, in addition, treated in individual psychotherapeutic sessions. At present systematic and intensive individual and group psychotherapy is also carried out in the neurotic department of the Psychiatric Research Institute in Prague. In the psychiatric hospital in Opava, besides individual and group psychotherapy, psychodramatic methods are used on a wide scale. At present there exists also a special psychotherapeutic subsection of the psychiatric association with regular meetings.

Other therapeutic methods that deserve attention are ergotherapy and occupational therapy, which are commonly used in mental hospitals and other psychiatric facilities and have reached a relatively high standard in some of them (Pezinok, Havlíckuv, Brod, etc.). Also musicotherapy, bibliotherapy, and arttherapy are used in some facilities as a supplement to other therapeutic methods.

Hydrotherapy and physiotherapy are found most often and used in treatment at spas. This form of treatment is highly developed in Czechoslovakia; and there are several balneological places where psychiatric patients predominantly are being treated (Jeseník, Dubí, Vráz, Vyšné Ruzbachy), most often after the termination of the basic therapeutic program which is handled at some other facility.

Special mention should be made of the Czechoslovak treatment of alcoholics and the anti-alcoholic service, which is among the best organized services in the world. The center of these activities is in the Psychiatric

---

* At present the psychoanalytical movement is represented by only a few members at large of the IPA who work in Prague.

Department of the Medical Faculty in Prague. Here the patients undergo a special everyday program, including deconditioning treatment, group psychotherapy, occupational therapy, cultural therapy, etc. This center maintains good and close cooperation with the emergency center for people intoxicated by alcohol. There also exist several other well-organized and well-equipped rehabilitation centers for alcoholics.

It can be stated in summary that there is in therapeutic endeavors in Czechoslovak psychiatry generally a trend toward treating the greatest possible number of patients as outpatients. Mental hospitals have undergone a far-reaching change toward humanization and socialization of the milieu and also toward a more human approach with patients. The prevailing practice is an all-out approach in which biological and psychological means of every kind are combined. Last but not least, much effort is directed toward popularization of modern psychiatric knowledge with the aim of eradicating the prejudices of the lay population against the mentally ill and of alleviating their condition after dismissal from psychiatric facilities.

CHAPTER SEVEN

Mental Health Services and Resources in Poland

BY
DR. TADEUSZ GNAT

HISTORICAL TRENDS

THE DEVELOPMENT OF POLISH PSYCHIATRY is closely connected with the history of the Polish nation. Until modern times the religious orders provided care for the mentally ill. Asylums and special institutions for the insane were first developed in the sixteenth century in Cracow. These came to be called *hospitale delirantium*. Records show that a center founded in Gdansk in the sixteenth century provided 358 beds with six wards for the insane. The first laws recognizing the insane as ill people and which were free of demonology were the Lithuanian Statutes of 1529.

At the end of the eighteenth century and the beginning of the nineteenth Poland lost her independence and was partitioned between Prussia, Russia, and Austria. When independence was regained in 1918, efforts were devoted to reconstruction and reorganization of the state apparatus. These included the integration of the health service. Plans were made for mental health care and for rebuilding of the many psychiatric institutions that had been destroyed during World War I. Health Services had previously been administered by different voluntary and private organizations.

The government now entrusted the administration and management of the health services to the General Management of Health Service in the Ministry of Internal Affairs (Home Office) and then (until the outbreak of World War II) to the Department of Health in the Ministry of Labor, Social Welfare and Health. The Polish Psychiatric Association, founded in 1920, exerted a great influence on the development and organization of the mental health service in the country. In 1925, there were forty-six psychiatric institutions with one psychiatric bed per 2,630 persons. As an auxiliary measure for the care of the mentally disturbed, the family-care program was established in Poland just before World War II. Eleven institutions acting in this field enlisted about 850 foster families, which took care of about 3,000 patients.

World War II was particularly disastrous for Poland and for Polish psychiatry: six million people, or one fifth of the population, perished during the war; 12,000 patients in psychiatric institutions died together with psychiatrists and other staff members. The great majority of mental hospitals were completely destroyed.

After World War II one of the first steps toward rebuilding the health services was to provide a social-insurance system for the public health services and facilities. Today, social insurance encompasses all the employed, and all payments toward social insurance are made exclusively by employers. The system provides free medical care and treatment, including mental health facilities: Drugs and doctors and other staff members are paid for, as are per diem costs of stay in hospitals and in special institutions and the costs of outpatient care and home assistance. Temporary money benefits are offered to the patients for a period not exceeding six months. These amount to 70 to 100 percent of the normal wage, depending on the family status of the insured and on whether he is treated at home, in a hospital, or in a sanitarium. When an alcoholic is the sole provider, his family is provided for during his compulsory treatment. In cooperation with the Union of Pensioners, Invalids and Retired and with the Commission for Invalids and Employment, whose task is the assessment of a person's working ability, the state insurance establishment pays invalid pensions to the mentally disabled, i.e., those suffering from schizophrenia, epilepsy, manic-depressive psychosis, etc.

The reconstruction of old or destroyed hospitals and clinics, the building of new ones, and the training of staff members were rapidly developed after World War II. The organization of psychiatric care and services was centralized in the Section for Nervous Diseases of the Ministry of Health.

The Institute of Psychoneurology and the Institute of Post-graduate Training of Physicians were established to support psychiatric research. In 1956 the Training Center for Clinical Psychology was established.

In spite of these considerable achievements the Polish mental health service still faces several difficult problems, such as the necessity of increasing the number of psychiatric beds and the number of well-trained personnel, and the interpretation of its legal responsibilities.

DEVELOPMENT OF THE MENTAL HYGIENE MOVEMENT

The mental hygiene movement in Poland started in 1930 when the Polish delegation took part in the Congress of Mental Hygiene held in Washington. In 1933 the Section of Mental Hygiene was established in the National Council of Health and given the task of coordinating the movement in Poland. In 1935 the Polish League of Mental Hygiene was organized and Dr. Oskar Bielawski began publishing the journal *Mental Hygiene*. At the same time, Dr. Kazimierz Dabrowski established the Institute of Mental Hygiene in Warsaw. Its aim was clinical and scientific research and popularization of mental hygiene principles. At the Institute the following units were organized: An inpatient department for neuropsychiatry; outpatient departments for neuroses, epilepsy, and speech and auditory disorders; logopedics for children; and an inpatient department for adult neurotics. The Institute also established courses and lectures for physicians, tutors, and nurses on mental hygiene problems and published the *Bulletin of Mental Hygiene*. Several local branches of the Institute were organized in various towns.

The general movement was halted by the beginning of World War II, but the Institute maintained its activities, concentrating its efforts on diminishing the psychological effects of war on the population and on the development of the outpatient departments for children and adults.

After the war, progress in these areas resumed its course. In 1949, mental hygiene activities were included in psychiatric-treatment institutions, and psychology was added to university curricula. In 1957, the activity of the Polish Mental Hygiene Society was resumed, and the Department of Mental Hygiene and Child Psychiatry of the Polish Academy of Sciences was established. The Department develops its scientific activity and the Polish Mental Hygiene Society popularizes the principles of mental hygiene through meetings, conferences, and lectures of both scientific and popular nature. The Department of Mental Hygiene and Child Psychiatry of the Polish Academy of Sciences bases its clinical training in the sanitarium for child neuropsychiatry in Sagorze near Warsaw.

CURRENT ADMINISTRATIVE PATTERNS

Psychiatric service in Poland is an integral part of the public health administration. Most of the mental health services are supervised by the Ministry of Health and Social Welfare. However, there are some branches subordinated to other ministries, such as the Ministry of Transport and the Ministry of National Defense. Because of the specific character of some psychiatric problems, the mental health service cooperates with the Ministry of Justice and the Ministry of Education. The assessment of working ability and the distribution of pensions is the responsibility of the Social Insurance Department. Mental health service is supervised by the Department of Prophylaxis and Therapeutics of the Ministry of Health, specifically by the Section for Nervous Diseases of this department.

The Ministry of Health and Social Welfare supervises the Institute of Psychoneurology, which plans, organizes, and carries out research in neurology, psychiatry, and allied branches. It coordinates the work of different scientific centers and institutions of public health and thus plays the role of the national specialist in psychiatry. In every district there is one chief psychiatrist named by the Ministry of Health and Social Welfare on the proposal of the Presidium of the District People's Council.

The local District Outpatient Mental Health Departments consist of specialized guidance centers, therapeutic units, laboratories for diagnostic purposes, general consultation offices, observation and therapeutic wards (up to 100 beds), and rehabilitation wards that provide work therapy in different workshops. These departments are administered locally by sections for organization and methodology, for registration, documentation, and statistics, as well as for budget and economy.

In addition to district departments there are county mental health departments which provide the following services: Specialized guidance centers, registration, documentation, and statistics sections, treatment rooms, and economy and budget sections.

Volunteer organizations—such as the Polish Red Cross, the Polish Committee of Social Relief, the League of Women, the Union of Pensioners, Invalid and Retired, the Union of the Deaf and Dumb, the Union of War Invalids, the Polish Union of the Blind, and the Society of Children's Friends—play an important role along with governmental "social protectors" in the organization and administration of social-relief services. Social protectors work as regular employees of the Department of Health and Social Welfare in the People's Councils. Their education consists of at least two years of vocational practice or secondary education and at least five years of vocational practice.

FINANCES

The expenses of organizing and managing the inpatient centers for treatment of nervous and mental diseases are paid from the governmental budget. Some centers are financed from the central budget and directly by the Ministry of Health and Social Welfare Departments at the District People's Councils.

The institutions for the treatment of nervous and mental diseases admit all patients who are in need of treatment regardless of their rights to free provisions. Hospitalization is free for the majority of the population— namely, for all working people who are insured. Those who are self-employed have to pay for their treatment. Care and treatment in the institutions are also free for retired people, disabled persons, students, and some professional groups (artists, and farmers whose average income is 12,200 zlotys* or less per year). Those who have no right to free provisions pay twenty zlotys per day of stay and treatment. This sum represents only 33 percent of the actual cost. Farmers whose average income exceeds 12,200 zlotys are among the paying group. Farmers grouped in production co-operatives pay fifteen zlotys per day, or 25 percent of the actual cost.

The outpatient mental health services are financed from the governmental budget.

SERVICE PROGRAMS

Mental patients who are acutely ill are directed to a psychiatric hospital. A certificate issued by the psychiatrist from an outpatient department or—in emergency cases—by any physician is needed for admission. For involuntary admission as well as for patients devoid of family care, the written consent of relatives or of a guardian is needed.

Due to the development of modern psychopharmacology the mean period of stay is about 100 days as compared to 300 days before World

* 1 zloty = approximately 4¢.

War II. Chronic mental patients able to work are admitted to the special rehabilitation and resocialization program. Work therapy and occupational therapy are the basic elements of the earliest stage of this program. It is parallel to the basic treatment in mental hospitals and sanitariums. Among the simplest forms of work therapy applied are recreation therapy and physical education, the objective being to stimulate activity. After the patient is sufficiently active, the occupational therapy begins. The choice of occupation is based on the special interest of the patient, his abilities, and the possibilities of his acquiring new forms of behavior and new habits through the performed occupation. Therapy is organized in the form of workshops. The outpatient therapy workshops present an intermediate stage between hospital workshops and the employment of the patient. The type of workshops operated depend on the regional manpower of the community as well as the possibilities of employment of patients in the shared-work establishments for the handicapped in industrial establishments after their discharge from the hospital.

The second stage of the rehabilitation program is the employment of the patient. Mental patients in Poland are employed by "sheltered-work" establishments and institutions organized by the Cooperative Movement of Work and of the Handicapped and Crippled People as well as by industrial institutions. The jobs performed in these establishments consist essentially of the simple, easy-to-learn and effective activities. These work establishments are each staffed with a physician, a psychiatrist, a psychologist, a nurse, and a social protector.

Another form of the sheltered-work program is cottage industry, which is based on the principle of close cooperation with the other forms of workshops and essentially is for the handicapped who for various reasons cannot go to the other establishments. There are also hotels established by the cooperative movement for the handicapped who do not have families.

In agricultural regions the treatment of patients is based on the family-care program, which consists of the personal care executed by selected families as well as the medical care provided by the nearest mental hospital. Such a system provides homelike conditions for the patient and makes possible agricultural activities for him. In this instance the hospital pays the foster family the equivalent per diem cost of hospitalization.

Mentally disturbed geriatric patients are admitted to the mental hospitals in emergency cases. Those suffering from senile dementia are transferred to special institutions after having attained remission. These institutions do not provide any active treatment. Some are managed by the Polish Catholics Association and are called "Caritas"; others are financed and administered by the government.

Mentally disturbed children and those with character disorders are placed under the care of children outpatient departments, neurological departments, and social-education centers. Children who need hospital treatment are placed in the children's wards of psychiatric hospitals and sanitariums for child neuropsychiatry, where there are primary schools and teaching programs.

Juvenile delinquents under seventeen years old, of both sexes, are subject to the decision of the juvenile-delinquency courts. Those with mitigated sentences are placed under guardianship. Educational and re-habilitation centers exist where pedagogic care as well as primary and vocational education are provided. The juvenile-delinquency courts may apply educational and rehabilitation measures such as admonition, parental supervision, guardianship, placement in educational institutions, and immediate or delayed placement in these rehabilitation centers.

Mentally retarded children and adolescents are evaluated with the cooperation of schools, parents, social-education centers, mental health centers, and neurological departments. Special selecting commissions pronounce the child's inability to learn at normal school and qualify him to go to special schools which provide obligatory school education and vocational education. Some of these schools are boarding schools and some are day schools. If in a given area there is no special school, special classes at normal primary schools are arranged. Severely mentally retarded children and adolescents who are not trainable are sent to the Special Aid Institutions which are sponsored by the government, or to the Caritas.

Polish anti-alcoholic legislation began in 1920 by providing partial restriction of the sale of alcoholic beverages and consumption. In 1956 the following social prescriptions were provided: Compulsory treatment of alcoholics, penalties for making habitual drinkers of minors, legal protection and care of habitual drinkers' families, and establishment of the "sober-down homes." Since alcoholism is recognized as a social plague, alcoholics are treated as patients in need of therapy. According to law the district authorities must run therapeutic institutions and the county and municipal authorities must support antialcoholic outpatient departments.

Compulsory institutional treatment of alcoholics is ordered by court for the habitual drinker who causes disintegration of his family and is a social nuisance. His stay in the institution cannot last more than two years.

After having passed the compulsory discontinuance treatment, he is directed to a rehabilitation or therapeutic establishment. Resocialization of the alcoholic is based on occupational therapy, whereby the patient carries out his previously acquired skills or learns a new activity. He is paid for his work, although it is primarily for therapeutic value.

The less severely disturbed alcoholic is treated on an outpatient basis, which consists of improvement of physical condition and discontinuance by pharmacological methods.

The sober-down homes were established in 1956 as emergency institutions as well as social organizations opposing alcohol addiction. They serve as detention homes for the drunk person disturbing public order. The alcoholic must pay for his stay there, which cannot exceed twenty-four hours.

Drug addiction in Poland is not a social problem. The few cases which have been attended were placed under supervision of mental health centers, and the addicts were then directed for discontinuance treatment to the psychiatric hospitals. Sexual offenders are sentenced to institutional confinement only if they are considered to be disorderly persons. Most cases of sexual deviation are treated as sexual neuroses.

Families with problems are welcomed to the Gamology outpatient department in the Institute of Mental Hygiene. However, this department mainly concerns itself with disturbances in the child-parent relationship.

Epilepsy in Poland is under the care of anti-epileptic outpatient departments at mental health centers. The care normally consists in continuous pharmacological treatment. In cases of acute disorder, patients are directed for hospital treatment to neurological or psychiatric inpatient departments. Epileptics able to work are employed in sheltered workshops or cooperatives for the handicapped.

Children suffering from *petit mal* attacks are treated in children's mental health centers as outpatients. Children with more severe cases of epilepsy are treated and educated in the sanitariums for child neuropsychology which maintain special schools for the mentally retarded epileptics and vocational schools.

New legal regulations may soon be adopted regarding admission to and discharge from mental hospitals. Under consideration are admission at the request of the patient or a relative of the patient or by court order with an accompanying medical certificate issued by the mental health administrative authorities. Currently, in emergency situations a patient may be admitted with the consent of his family.

Discharge may be effected by the director of a hospital under the following conditions: If the patient is recovered, or if he can be treated at home, or if he is still in need of treatment but is not dangerous to himself or to the community.

RESEARCH

The Polish Psychiatric Association was established to coordinate the research in social psychiatry. A special conference on research programs and methods was held in Lublin in 1961 and laboratories of social psychiatry were established in Cracow and Warsaw. A number of widespread works in epidemiology were conducted by psychiatrists, psychologists, and sociologists dealing mainly with mental disease and mental deficiency, alcoholism, neurosis, and suicide. Attention was focused on large cities such as Cracow and newly organized industrial centers.

TRAINING

The psychiatry training program covers general psychopathology and clinical psychiatry as well as therapy of mental diseases. Fifth-year students of the medical academies are taught the basic knowledge of psychiatry in the course of sixty hours of lectures and thirty hours of practical training. Emphasis is placed on the method of case presentation as illustration to the lectures. Recently, training has included all problems connected with psychoneuroses and psychosomatic medicine with focus on the links between psychiatry and other specialties and the inter-dependency of psychiatry and social structures. The programs for medicine and psychiatry may soon be increased in scope and hours.

Psychiatry has been a medical specialty separated from neurology since 1953. This specialization is supported by the Institute for Postgraduate Training of Physicians through grants and scholarships, which are awarded on the basis of application. There are two grades of specialization for which postgraduate physicians can train in adult and child psychiatry. Training takes place in the psychiatric clinics of the ten medical academies in Poland and in the Institute of Psychoneurology in Pruszkow. Specialized training for postgraduates in psychiatry is conducted in psychiatric hospitals and includes two stages: The first stage consists of three years experience in clinical practice and the passing of an examination administered at the district health department. This includes psychiatric examination and diagnosis of case reports; interpretation of different laboratory findings; basic information on drugs and various therapeutic methods; techniques of psychiatric therapy and child psychiatry; problems of neuroses and their treatment, with emphasis placed on psychotherapy; alcoholism and aftercare of alcoholic patients; and acquaintance with medical indications for hospitalization and sanitarium treatment.

A candidate for the title of Specialist in psychiatry for adults must prove to be acquainted with the organization of hospital work, the principles of forensic observation in mental hospitals, and the duties of a psychiatric expert in court procedures. He is trained in methods of examination of neurological and internal disease and acquainted with the diagnosis of borderline cases. The training program also includes study of pathological anatomy of the central nervous system.

The training program for the Second Grade Specialist in adult psychiatry comprises diagnostic and therapeutic problems including laboratory tests, the principles of clinical psychology, psychotherapy, work therapy, and biological treatment methods. The candidate for the Second Grade should be familiar with modern psychiatric conceptions, legal regulations concerning the mentally ill, alcoholics, drug addicts, psychiatric staff, problems of social psychiatry, and pathological anatomy with particular emphasis placed on anatomy of the human brain and the achievement of modern neurophysiology. In addition the candidate is expected to have a firm knowledge of forensic psychiatry, child psychiatry, clinical treatment and therapy of neuroses including psychotherapy, some problems of general medicine directly connected with psychiatry, and basic information about clinical neurology.

The duration of the postgraduate training (partial training) in clinical disciplines interrelated with psychiatry (internal diseases, neurology, forensic psychiatry, and child psychiatry) is not strictly determined by any regulation and is to be defined in every case by the specialist responsible for the training. After twenty-four months of postgraduate clinical training (or training in a hospital, which must be supplemented by three months of training at a psychiatric clinic or at the Psychoneurological Institute) the candidate is obliged to pass an examination in the appropriate medical academy before a board consisting of at least two independent scientists (professors, assistant professors, and docents). The number of specialized psychiatrists (First and Second Grade) has increased from 177 in 1952 to 518 in 1962.

A Second Grade specialization in child psychiatry is now being introduced. The First Grade specialization in psychiatry or pediatrics is required from a candidate. The training schedule embraces twelve months of internship in social and clinical pediatrics, six months in child neurology, anad fifteen months of internship at the psychiatric ward for children. Courses in clinical and educational psychology are also obligatory. The First Grade Specialists in pediatrics are obliged to spend a six-month internship in psychiatric wards for adults, eighteen months in a psychiatric ward for children, and three months in a neurological ward for children. Courses in clinical and educational psychology are also required. In both cases the minimum time of training necessary to obtain a specialization grade in child psychiatry is thirty-six months (including three months of vacation).

The Institute of the Postgraduate Training of Physicians offers courses and nonresident training in all the disciplines of medicine including psychiatry. Thematic training includes specialized courses, national and international seminars and conferences, lectures, and clinical rounds. For the physicians from outside Warsaw special courses (nonresident courses) have been organized. Their aim is to acquaint the physicians with essential medical problems.

Local units of the Polish Psychiatric Association organize monthly meetings devoted to the problems of diagnosis and therapy. Individual sections of this association (for example, the Psychotherapy section) also organize monthly seminars for nonresidents.

The university curriculum in psychology extends over five years and leads to an M.A. degree granted upon completion of a written dissertation and an examination. Clinical psychology is one of several fields of specialization in psychology and is offered for study at the Universities of Warsaw, Cracow, and Poznan, and at the Catholic University of Lublin.

A training center for clinical psychology was established in 1956 in the laboratory of clinical psychology in the State Hospital for Nervous and Mentally Ill in Cracow-Kobierzyn. This center offers practical training in psychological diagnosis.

PSYCHOLOGY

More than 200 psychologists staff psychiatric hospitals including those for neurological disorders, pediatrics and tuberculosis. Although psychologists and psychiatrists cooperate there is still discussion on the role of the

psychologist in the process of psychotherapy. Many psychiatrists assume
that only physicians can undertake the responsibility of psychotherapy. At
present the regulations concerning the professional work of psychologists
in mental health service are being worked out and a resolution concerning
this is being prepared by the Polish Psychological Association.

Most psychologists are trained in psychotheraphy in special courses
for physicians and psychologists organized by the Polish Psychiatric Association. The Ministry of Health and Social Welfare established in 1966
the Postgraduate Training Center for Clinical Psychologists. Its program
comprises diagnosis, psychotheraphy, and rehabilitation of mentally ill
children and adults. The duration of internship is set at two years.

At the Polish Academy of Sciences Psychometrical Laboratory there
exists a small clinical-psychology unit supported by the Ministry of Health
and Social Welfare. This unit is working on adaptation and standardiza-
tion of tests for clinical use.

Group therapy is conducted at the Center for Treatment of Neuroses
at Rasztow by one physician, two psychologists, and one nonmedical person. All psychotherapists have undergone at least one year of training as
observers or participants in small therapeutic groups. But the basic condition for becoming a psychotherapist is the person's own training analysis
which enables him to have an insight into his individual problems, control
his attitude toward patients, and limit his own emotional traits in the interpretation of patients' personalities. All psychotherapists at the Center work
independently, but play similar roles.

In order to promote mental health in Poland, an effort is being made
to propagate psychiatric knowledge beyond the professional groups. Various
forms of mental health training have been organized for representatives
of other professions who in their work have contact with the mentally ill.
Seminars on mental hygiene devoted to the training of teachers are organized by the Ministry of Education and conducted by the Institute for
the Postgraduate Training of Physicians. Specialized teachers employed
in schools for retardates are trained at the Institute of Special Pedagogics.
Educational conferences dealing with problems of psychic and nervous
disturbances including child neuroses and prevention of mental diseases
are organized by the Polish Academy of Sciences for psychologists and
general practitioners. Lectures and short conferences for psychologists and
sociologists employed in industry are given by the Labor Section for
Mental Hygiene.

Two-year medical schools for instructors in occupational therapy at psychiatric hospitals in Branice and Toszek opened in 1962 and now graduate about sixty students per year. The schools admit candidates who have completed secondary schooling.

Instructors in physical training are usually graduated from the Warsaw Academy of Physical Training or another university school of this type. They participate in recreation therapy. Kinesitherapists trained in special two-year schools have similar tasks. There are two schools for kinesitherapists subordinate to kinesitherapy centers in Poznan and Konstancin near Warsaw.

CHAPTER EIGHT

Development, Current Status, and Prospects of Bulgarian Psychiatry

BY
DR. I. TEMKOV AND DR. I. STOIMENOV

FOUNDED IN THE YEAR 681, the Bulgarian state early reached a high level of intellectual and material development. Because of its geography, it came under the influence of Greek, Roman, Byzantine, Thracian, Slavic, and other cultures. Bulgaria has been under both the Byzantine yoke (1018–1185) and the Turkish yoke (1396–1878). It was liberated from Turkish domination by Russia, after a prolonged and heroic revolutionary struggle.

A decisive turning point in the development of Bulgaria was reached after September 9, 1944, when the country, with the resolute help of the Soviet army, freed itself from fascism and set off energetically on the road of its socialist construction.

In conformity with the principal stages in the development of Bulgaria, it is proper to divide the history of Bulgarian psychiatry into three periods:

1. Up to liberation from Turkey (1878)
2. After liberation from Turkey to September 9, 1944
3. From September 9, 1944, to today.

Until the liberation, Turkish domination played a catastrophic role, not only because of the obliteration of any organization of medical aid but also owing to the feudal conditions of economic oppression, poverty, and obscurantism in the Turkish Empire. Because of these factors, the intellectual and economic development of Bulgaria was reduced to zero.

Beginning in the ninth century—the so-called "golden century" of Bulgarian culture—the natural science that originated in Byzantium was disseminated throughout Slavic and Western European countries. In that century, John the Exarch wrote *The Heavens* and *The Hexameron*, in which human anatomy, psychology, and personality are examined. Thus, a large forehead was thought to indicate a sagacious intellect; a small one, sharper wits; a broad brow, cowardice; and a round one, an importunate, impatient, and angry character.

The epistle of the Patriarch Euthymious (fourteenth century) focused cn psychosexual problems such as masturbation and homosexuality and advised various hygienic and social measures against them, such as, "that masturbation may be forgiven, but homosexuals and those who indulge in sodomy should not be ordained as clergymen."

Aid to the mentally ill in this period was rendered by the monasteries, sorcerers, and exorcisers. The mentally ill were given asylum in the Bachkovski Monastery near Asenovgrad, the Monastery of St. George in the city of Nevrokop, the Monastery of St. Naum near Lake Okhrid, and the Rilski Monastery, Khrel'ova Castle.

During the Bulgarian renaissance, conditions for cultural revival were created, and a number of young men went off to study in foreign countries. Many of them did not return to Bulgaria, and there was little development of knowledge in the natural sciences and little penetration of medical knowledge or therapeutic practice among the Bulgarian people. Views on the causes, onset, and development of mental illness continued to be of a mystical, religious character, and the treatment of the mentally ill continued to be carried out in monasteries and sanctuaries by monks, Turkish priests (imams), or Jewish clergymen (rabbis). Popular medicine also operated through spells, exorcisms, and other religious and mystical rituals.*

---

* In the nineteenth century, medical books began to be published in Bulgaria. These books were not scientific but presented translations of popular articles from Russian or Western periodicals. An example of the type of book published is Zakhariia Kniazheski's *Lectures on Drunkenness and the Relief It Affords to Those Who Drink a Lot* (Smyrna, 1842) in which people who abuse alcohol are criticized, and the consequences for physical and mental health are pointed out. Among the

The second period in the development of Bulgarian psychiatry began with the liberation from Turkey in 1878. The demolished feudal structure was replaced by a structure of small, independent commodity producers in the towns and in the country. These followed a period of initial capital accumulation and the creation and expansion of industrial production. By the end of the nineteenth century, the newly constituted big bourgeoisie took over the leadership of the country from the petty bourgeoisie. The principal resources and know-how of the state went into the construction of roads, railways, and ports and the arming of troops for the aggressive purposes of Bulgarian capitalism. The health of the people was relegated to the background.

There were, however, some developments in medicine because of the efforts, patriotism and sense of social duty of a few physicians who came from the milieu of the petty bourgeoisie but who had completed their medical education in Russia.* Influenced by progressive Zemstvo medicine, they advocated medical assistance and prophylaxis for the general working population.

The first special psychiatric department in Bulgaria—in Sofia, at the Aleksandrovska Hospital—was opened in 1888. In 1902, in two old buildings near the Karlukovo station, an insane asylum was opened—originally with thirty-two beds, increased later to eighty-eight beds. Eight years later, in the city of Biala in Northern Bulgaria, another insane asylum was opened in an abandoned Turkish barracks. This was rebuilt as a hospital in 1929. The psychiatric network later came to include departments in the Khaskovo and Razgrad Hospitals and the Balbunar Asylum for epileptics in the town of Kotel.

This was all accomplished prior to World War I. From that time until September 9, 1944, the only construction was of the neuropsychiatric clinic of the medical faculty in Sofia with 200 beds. Until then, the number of beds and the conditions in psychiatric establishments and asylums were quite inadequate. Supplies and personnel were scarce, and the application of active methods of treatment limited. Occupational therapy

---

popular articles printed in the first Bulgarian periodical, *Liuboslovie* (Literary Curiosities), published in 1844–1847 by the celebrated leader of the Bulgarian National Revival, Konstantin Fotinov, were some in medicine and natural science. For example, "The Human Brain," contains data on the structure and functions of the brain. In 1872, in the periodical *Chitalishte* (Reading-Room), "A Note on Melancholia" was published. A more serious work is the dissertation by Dr. P. Selvili, "On the Pathoanatomy of Paralytic Dementia," published in Zurich (Switzerland) in 1876.

* D. Molov, P. Orakhovatz, and others.

and psychotherapy were only occasionally administered. Prior to September 9, 1944, only twenty persons in Bulgaria were recognized as specialists in neurology and psychiatry.

However, good results were achieved in a number of psychiatric hospitals because of the devotion of some outstanding psychiatrists. One such person was Georgi Paiakov, who directed a hospital in Lovech, Northern Bulgaria. Reporting on the hospital's work (1910), he wrote:

> When I began to equip the department, I attempted to introduce, as far as this was possible, modern methods for the care of the mentally ill, guided by the idea that medicine is not the only important element in the cure of the mentally ill, but also good surroundings, unreserved, kind and humane care . . . The open door is an ideal of modern psychiatry and much has been accomplished in this respect . . . The aim was to make the atmosphere of the department approximate that in the home. Flowers and pictures have been introduced. The patients have been provided with various games: dominoes, cards. An exception is made for patients who damage these things. A phonograph with many new records was bought, and also books, newspapers, and magazines. . .

After the construction of the first psychiatric departments and the advent of physicians specializing in psychiatry certain modest conditions were created for scientific work.* The principal activity in this period was the organization of neuropsychiatric clinics.

Although the major influence came from German psychiatry, the effect of classical Russian—and also Soviet—psychiatry was intensified during this time. The Russian influence came primarily through the activity of the Russian professors N. M. Popov and A. E. Yanshevski, who headed the psychiatry and neurology clinics in the first Bulgarian Faculty of Medicine in Sofia which was founded in 1918.† The Soviet influence derived from the school of the great Russian physiologist, I. P. Pavlov.

Popov was concerned with the multiple etiology of progressive paralysis (syphilis and various other exo- and endotoxic influences on the nervous system). In his study of congenital epilepsy, he stressed the importance of social factors and living conditions as well as of alcohol and cranial injuries.

The materialistic direction of Bulgarian psychiatry was represented by Nikola Gavrilov Krustnikov (1880–1936), who was the first Bulgarian

---

* The most prominent psychiatrists were S. Danadzhiev, G. Paiakov, V. Vladov, D. Kalevich, D. Barakov, A. Golovina, N. Moskov, and M. Mikhailov.

† N. Popov was the author of the first Bulgarian textbooks on psychiatry, *Fundamentals of General Psychopathology* (1923), and *Fundamentals of Special Psychopathology* (1925). These emphasized the principals of German idealistic psychiatry and stressed clinical problems, especially progressive paralysis and schizophrenia.

teacher of psychiatry. In opposition to the idealistic trend in psychiatry, Krustnikov perceived the material bases of psychic life to be reflex activity. The nucleus of his scientific studies is represented by his *The Psychon Doctrine** and by his studies of psychic life in normal and pathological conditions.

He differentiated the simple reflex activity of the spinal cord and the lower centers from that nervous activity which underlies psychic life:

> The process of perception is a psychic act, even though it derives in principle from reflexes, i.e., has as its basis the anatomical and physiological characteristics of the reflex neuron, but since, in the case of perception, the latter already belongs to a different category, in terms of function, we shall therefore designate it for greater clarity, as a psychon.

The elementary functional units of psychic activity were, then, "psychons," which correspond to neurons in nervous activity. At the center of all psychons is an "ego psychon," "a central point in the conscious processes," around which all other centrifugal and centripetal psychons are ranged. Later, Krustnikov assigned to each psychon a "sensitive psychon," uniting the centrifugal and centripetal psychons into a single psychon with a centrifugal and a centripetal part. Psychic life was seen as the result of reflex processes among an "ego psychon" and the other psychons, and psychic disorders as the result of derangement of the centrifugal and centripetal reflex activity of the psychons.

With these concepts he examined particular psychic processes and psychopathological states and also the existence of consciousness. Thus, for example, perception, according to Krustnikov, is made up of two psychons: a centripetal one (sensory, perceptual) and a centrifugal one (representational). Of the conscious processes, he writes:

> The organized psychon, which is basically the sum of the sensations of the physical organs (internal organs, muscles, joints, etc.), represents a central point for mental life, a sort of main focus for the conscious processes . . . The process of perception itself . . . so long as it is not connected with "ego" perception, is merely a physiological process—an unconscious act.

Thus, as the cause of various disturbances of consciousness, Krustnikov sees changes in the state of the ego psychon (the sphere of physical sensations and mental representations); this may, for example, be suppression or anesthetization of the links between it and the other psychons. If the suppression involves both centripetal psychons and the centrifugal

---

* This doctrine was elaborated in *Toward a Doctrine of the Basic Principles of the Mental Processes* (1924), *Physical Sensations and Conscious Processes* (1926), and *The Principle of Dissociation in Neurology and Psychiatry* (1934).

ego psychon, complete loss of consciousness is observed, with total amnesia; in the case of suppression of the centrifugal ego psychon only, a sleeping state occurs, with automatism and partial amnesia. In some cases, total amnesia is caused by anasthesia of the links between the ego psychon and the other psychons. However, under the influence of affects, the links between an ego psychon and the other psychons may be pathologically excited. This phenomenon underlies obsessive ideas.

Krustnikov considered hallucinations to be the result of pathological excitation of the corresponding centripetal psychons and attributed pseudo-hallucinations to excitation in the centrifugal psychons.

In 1934, Krustnikov published his work *The Principle of Dissociation in Neurology and Psychiatry.* Starting from the concept of dissociation of functions in the nervous system, introduced by Head and Riddoch, Krustnikov developed it in neuropathology and psychopathology. He formulated this principle as follows: "Dissociation in neuropathology and psychopathology deals with the capacity of individual nerves and psychic functions to acquire an autonomous—we would add, heightened—activity. This independent existence constitutes the main feature of dissociation."

The heightened activity of the dissociated systems he conceives as a manifestation of active defense, designed to reestablish the previous links. Krustnikov gives an original explanation of the symptoms of excitation: he considers that what we call irritative symptoms are due not to damage to the nervous system but to dissociation of undamaged systems. This is why, in a pathological process, one must look for lost or weakened functions; they reflect primarily damaged nervous systems, whereas the symptoms of excitation and irritation are secondary.

These theoretical positions were given concrete form by Krustnikov in the elucidation of a number of symptoms and syndromes in psychiatry. Thus, for example: "In mania, there are tyrannical, deafening, unpleasant feeling tones, manifested in inordinately heightened asthenic emotions, but the mechanism must be regarded as the result of weakened or lost function of the pleasant feeling tones, while the functions of the asthenic tones are still operative."

In formulating the problems of the dissociation of functions in neuropathology and psychopathology, Krustnikov exhibited a tendency to relate psychopathological manifestations to physiological processes, such as those described by I. P. Pavlov. He writes:

Clinical observation shows us that in the subject correlation of an excitatory and an inhibitory process, we see clearly that they correspond to certain psychic processes. That is to say, an excitatory process is accompanied by predominant functioning of unpleasant feeling tones. And in the physiological experiments of Pavlov, the same regular correlation is obtained which clinical observation also yields us. Thus, the results of psychopathological analysis closely approximate the results of neurophysiological analysis with respect to the primitively confused functions in mania and melancholia.

A number of psychotic symptoms and syndromes, like psychic automatism or suggestibility (echolalia, echopraxia, hypnosis, flexibilitas cerea, etc.), Krustnikov also regarded as being due to loss of the two functions referred to above, and in an affective state, ". . . there is always a weakening or lack of one of the functions basic to psychic activity: either the functioning of pleasant tones or that of unpleasant tones."

He sought to discover the basic disorders in psychoses. Thus, in schizophrenia, he considered the primarily disturbed functions to be the loss of a sense of logic (lack of perception of the operation of the thinking process) and of the sensation of psychic activity. Here, too, Krustnikov makes an effort to relate the weakened sensation of activity to the weakening of the "purposive reflex," after Pavlov.

Starting from his theoretical understanding of the regularities in psychic activity and of the basic etiopathogenic mechanisms in the development of neurotic conditions, Krustnikov devised and promulgated his original psychotherapeutic method in *The Therapeutic Effect of Artificially Provoked Reproduction of Pathogenic Experiences* (1929). Placed in a recumbent position, the patient reproduces his psychologically traumatic experiences in three successive stages: First, the so-called "organic group" (physical changes); after that, the emotional content of the experiential-emotional group; and lastly, the sensory-perceptual group—the objective content of the affective experience. Repeated reproductions lead, in most cases, to beneficial therapeutic results.

Although the reproduction method belongs, in essence, among the methods of psychocatharsis, it excels all similar methods developed before it because, above all, it achieves a condition that approximates the natural one, as the suggestive influence of the physician is reduced to a minimum.

The method of Krustnikov was favorably received, not only in Bulgaria, but in the international literature as well. There were a number of enthusiastic reviews from such scholars as Vogt and Stoerring. Stoerring, in comparing it with other psychotherapeutic methods, considers that its advantage as against Frank's psychocatharsis is ascribable to the elimination of hypnosis and even of a hypnoid state, and also, to the limitation of medical intervention and suggestion to the least possible extent. In relation to the psychoanalytic method of Freud, Stoerring sees N. Krustnikov's as superior in its avoidance both of hypnosis and of frequently repeated interpretation of the morbid symptoms. Thus, according to Stoerring, the reproduction method of Krustnikov is the best of the psychotherapeutic methods and comes closest to the experimental methods for the revelation and explication of human emotional life.

An ardent adherent of the psychotherapeutic ideas of Krustnikov was Dr. E. Shekhanova (1899–1962). Her best-known work is the Psychoneuroses as a *Key to the Endogenous Psychoses in the Light of Analytical Psychiatry and the New Therapeutic Methods* (1942). Another celebrated psychiatrist in this period was Dr. Kh. Petrov (1901–1944), who, unhappily, perished during the bombardment of Sofia. He worked mainly on the problems of general psychopathology. His studies on schizophrenia were *Catatonia and Higher Nervous Activity* (1934), and *The Pathophysiology of Catatonic Stupor* (1938).

During the years when the country was dominated by fascism, the basic orientation in scientific research was clinical, and its sole methods were clinical analysis and clinical-statistical analysis. Clinical-experimental and purely experimental methods were scarcely employed at all. As far as methodology was concerned, Bulgarian psychiatry, in its fundamental tendencies, was based for the most part on idealistic positions and was persuaded into a number of reactionary theories (Lombroso's typology, "Neo-Lombrosism," German criminal biology, etc.).

During this period monarcho-fascist literature was also prevalent in Bulgaria, especially after the rapprochement of the bourgeoisie in Hitler's Germany. This resulted in the development of some pseudoscientific theories and misanthropic racist ideas among some psychiatrists.* Unfortunately, the celebrated Bulgarian morphologist, neurologist, and psychiatrist, Professor A. Penchev, who had done outstanding work on tellurism, lead poisoning, and pellagrous psychoses, also defended harsh racist views. He was an adherent of the "grading" of citizens "from the standpoint of their intellectual and ethnic value as assessed by psychiatrists." As a result of these concepts, A. Penchev came to the conclusions that it was necessary to introduce a sterilization law.†

---

* Representatives of these tendencies were Dr. R. Rusev, *Basic Criteria of Eugenic–Racial Hygiene* (1934) and Dr. I. Antonov, *Criminal Biology in the Service of Combating and Preventing Crime in Germany*, in which the positions of German criminal biology are defended.

† *On the Neuropsychiatric Field in Bulgaria* (1941).

During the Second World War, the Bulgarian fascist power, embittered by popular opposition, increasingly neglected the country's health problems. The Ministry of National Health, inquiring into conditions at the hospital in Biala after the liberation, reported:

A foul reek and chill exhalation rises from the huge halls, filled to overflowing with patients, some of them clothed in rags, and others, completely naked, piled one against the other, and on top of the other, forming towers of naked human bodies. The patients' bodies are emaciated, with scabies and louse wounds. The beds, such as they are, are without sheets, with bare straw mattresses and one threadbare blanket each. There are no eating utensils, and rusty cans are used instead of glasses. On the ringing of a railway bell, all the patients go down into the cellar, where the dining room is located. . . .

Outpatient psychiatric care in Bulgaria before September 9, 1944, was carried out by a small number of neurologists and psychiatrists who practiced privately in Sofia's neuropsychiatric clinic and in a few provincial psychiatric hospitals.

Subsequent to the war, basic reforms were brought about in economic, political and cultural life, and the national health services were completely reshaped. The organization of psychiatric treatment which occurred at this time was influenced by the organization of Soviet psychiatry. From this time on the guiding principals of outpatient treatment were those of prophylaxis and mental hygiene. After considerable study of various organizational patterns, the first neuropsychiatric dispensaries,* modeled after those in the U.S.S.R., were established in 1951. Although in existence for only about thirteen years, they are today the nucleus of practical psychiatric activity.

After September 9, 1944, Bulgarian psychiatric science was confronted with a number of fundamental tasks. First came the effort to develop a staff of good scientists and science teachers and to give them theoretical training based on progressive international and Soviet psychiatric science. Parallel with this task, attention was directed to the creation of new institutions for scientific research and of clinical centers. Of no small importance was the assessment of problems of scientific research through conferences, discussions, scientific meetings, and examinations of monographs and other scientific publications.

A fundamental role was played by discussions on the basic method-

---

* Although they are called "neuropsychiatric," in terms of their actual work, they are primarily psychiatric, since they deal with the investigation, prevention, and treatment of mental diseases. The neurological organization is set up separately in the system of hospitals and outpatient units for somatic diseases.

ological problems of neurology and psychiatry, held in 1949 at the Faculty of Medicine in Sofia. The principal address was delivered by G. Uzunov. It constituted a broad theoretical platform and on the basis of it a number of erroneous tendencies in the methodology of Bulgarian psychiatry were scrutinized. At the same time, prospects for its development were mapped out. A new and even broader survey of the status and tasks of Bulgarian psychiatry was undertaken by the First National Conference on Bulgarian Neurology and Psychiatry (1954), at which the theoretical and actual status of Bulgarian psychiatry was assessed on the basis of a critical report delivered by I. Temkov.

Of immense importance are the national conferences—six to date— held every two years. Here Bulgarian psychiatrists and neurologists discuss important scientific and political organizational problems: new trends in the organization of Bulgarian psychiatry, problems of rehabilitation and psychotherapy, psychopharmacologic problems, etc. The decisions and resolutions adopted constitute a basic document which determines the main stages of the development of psychiatric theory and practice for a period of two years. The active participation and cooperation of the Ministry of National Health in these conferences ensures the implementation of the decisions made.

The methodological formulation of the decisions made of Bulgarian psychiatry was accomplished both through the specialization of physicians in the U.S.R.R. and through the enormous amount of Soviet psychiatric literature which was introduced into our country and used, in fistfuls, by Bulgarian psychiatrists.

A very important factor in the development of Bulgarian psychiatry was the expansion of the system of scientific research establishments in the field of psychiatry. Until 1944, the sole scientific psychiatric institution was the neuropsychiatric clinic of the Faculty of Medicine in Sofia. After this date a number of establishments were opened.* A leading role in this activity was played by the Faculty of Medicine in Sofia, under the direction of Professor G. Uzunov. He actively worked to develop the clinical-experimental and purely experimental approaches, coordination of psychiatry with neurology and other medical sciences, rapid and thorough

---

* Department of Psychiatry at the Faculty of Medicine in Plovdiv (Southern Bulgaria): Scientific Research Institute of Neurology and Psychiatry in the Ministry of National Health (Sofia); Department of Psychiatry at the Institute for Specialization and Postgraduate Training of Physicians (Sofia); scientific group for neurology and psychiatry at the Bulgarian Academy of Sciences; and, in 1961, Department of Psychiatry at the Faculty of Medicine in Varna (Eastern Bulgaria).

equipping of psychiatric establishments with modern apparatus and methodological reorganization of Bulgarian psychiatry on the basis of Soviet and international progressive psychiatric science in opposition to idealism and speculative theories in clinical psychiatry.

G. Uzunov has done creative work on the clinical aspects and pathology of intoxication of the nervous system (atabrine, bromine, luminal [phenobarbital], alcohol) and on encephalitides, principally the so-called "subacute progressive hyperkinetic encephalitis." With S. Bozhinov, he described a new clinical and pathomorphologic form of acute alcoholism in childhood, characterized by bilateral softening of the putamen. His experimental studies established the role of the vasoreceptors of the pulmonary circulation in the development of epileptiform attacks. He also studied reactivity in chronic schizophrenia and epilepsy.

An active part in the development of Bulgarian psychiatric science was also taken by the group of the psychiatric clinic in the city of Plovdiv. Its director, Professor K. Cholakov (1897–1963), worked outside academic circles before September 9, 1944, and published a number of works on the neuroses, psychopathies, etc. Of considerable interest is his original psychotherapeutic method which he called "psychophysiological decapsulation as a causal treatment of neuroses." After 1944, he worked on problems of general psychopathology, epilepsy, etc. With his group of young co-workers, he also investigated problems of psychotherapy and neuroses and conducted clinical experimental studies on medical psychology and the role of barrier mechanisms in the pathogenesis and therapy of some mental illnesses.

In the last ten years psychopharmacologic studies have formed the nucleus of modern experimental psychiatry in a number of clinics. The sound traditions of forensic psychiatry already formulated by S. Danadzhiev were explained and raised to a contemporary level. The works of Professor N. Schipkowensky on responsibility and irresponsibility, forensic psychiatric problems in schizophrenia, manic-depressive psychosis, and oligophrenia were of major importance.

Child psychiatry has also occupied a prominent place. Up to September 9, 1944, one of the few people active in this field was Dr. V. Shumanov, who dealt mainly with questions of medical pedagogy and of neurotic illnesses in childhood. Today, this branch of psychiatry in Bulgaria has developed quite rapidly. Interesting recent studies in this field have been published by Kh. Khristov. V. Ionchev, L. Dzhartov, M. Gulubova, M. Achkova, N. Dashinova, and others.

Serious theoretical, methodological, and practical development has been attained in the organization of psychiatry and in the related field of investigation of the epidemiology of mental illnesses. The problems of the organization of the psychiatric setup, of the clinic system in the field of psychiatry, and of the distribution of mental illnesses in Bulgaria, have been worked out.* Also, sound bases have been laid for the purposeful resolution of complex problems. Scientific specialties have been carved out in the narrowest fields of scientific research. Years of investigation devoted to particular problems have made possible the writing of larger works of the monograph type as well as the publication of separate collections and manuals on related problems.

Individual institutes or clinics are now each concerning themselves primarily with a selected group of problems. Thus, for example, the neurology and psychiatry group in the Bulgarian Academy of Sciences is working on the changes in encephalitis from an experimental standpoint; the psychopharmacology group in the Department of Psychiatry of the Faculty of Medicine in Sofia, on a number of problems of exogenous-toxic psychoses; a group at the Scientific Research Institute of Neurology and Psychiatry, on the clinical aspects and pathophysiology of schizophrenia; the Department of Psychiatry at Plovdiv, on the problems of forensic psychiatry. These problems are approached by means of clinical, biochemical, electroencephalographic, histological, virological, radioisotrope, and various additional methods of investigation in combination with each other.

Groups in the peripheral psychiatric hospitals and clinics are also taking part in scientific work. They study the outpatient treatment of the psychoses and make catamnestic studies of treatment with psychopharmacologic agents, for example.

Today, Bulgarian psychiatry is facing a new stage in its development. It is confronted with the task of providing rapid training for growing numbers of highly qualified personnel in the various branches of scientific study—histochemistry, biochemistry, electrophysiology, medical genetics, experimental psychology and psychiatry, etc.—who will be the indispensable collaborators of the clinicians. Another aspect of this new era is the growing tendency for much closer coordination and cooperation in scientific research work among the individual institutes and laboratories. This should ensure against preoccupation with unimportant problems and undesirable duplication as well as promote elaboration of scientific studies on the highest level.

Scientific work has been stimulated, from the social standpoint, by

* See References 6, 7, 8, 9, 19, 20, 22, and 25.

the Association of Bulgarian Neurologists, Psychiatrists, and Neuro-surgeons, which is an association common to all physicians in the country and has individual branches in the large cities. Within the Republic-wide association, some more narrowly delimited sections have also been formed: of clinical electrophysiology, of psychotherapy, of forensic medicine, and of sexual pathology. The Association and its sections organize scientific meetings and national conferences and encourage participation in the international congresses and symposia. Concrete proposals for improving the organization of scientific and practical activity in psychiatry are sub-mitted to the Ministry of Health. The Association participates in the dissemination of scientific knowledge among the people, chiefly with respect to psychoprophylaxis and mental hygiene, the public war on alcoholism and delinquency in children. It also helps in the organization of educational programs, especially in schools for psychopathic and oligo-phrenic children. Its organ is the journal *Neurology, Psychiatry, and Neurosurgery,* which publishes scientific papers in these fields. The association gets economic assistance from the Ministry of National Health and moral support and cooperation from various social organizations.

There are thirteen neuropsychiatric clinics in Bulgaria today, cor-responding to the administrative divisions of the country as of 1951–1952. Each clinic serves from 300,000 to 800,000 people and comprises two important functionally unified units—the outpatient section, with spe-cialized consulting rooms, and the inpatient unit. A clinic is directed by a highly qualified specialist in psychiatry.

In the outpatient section, besides a general psychiatric consulting room, there are consulting rooms for child psychiatry, forensic psychiatry, psychotherapy, narcotherapy, neurology, and speech therapy. Special physicians, all psychiatrists, work in each of these consulting rooms.

The inpatient units of the neuropsychiatric clinics have between thirty and seventy beds, which are used primarily for diagnostic work and the treatment of mild disorders not in need of psychiatric hospital treatment, such as neuroses and psychopathies.

The neuropsychiatric clinics receive direction from the Ministry of National Health and Social Affairs as regards organization and personnel; from the departments of National Health and Social Affairs of the Regional People's Councils, as regards personnel, finances, and economics; and from the Scientific Research Institute of Neurology and Psychiatry with respect to methodological and scientific problems. A clinic is, also, in close contact with the district health services, polyclinics, hospitals for somatic illness, and psychiatric hospitals.

These clinics are the outposts of the psychiatric organization. Through them, psychiatric treatment is brought as close to the population as possible. This decentralized method of specialized service to the population (not only in psychiatry, but also in other types of medical treatment) undoubtedly is conducive to fuller and earlier detection of disease as well as to better treatment. I. Stoimenov and his coworkers found that there is an inverse relationship between the rate of mental illness and the distance from neuropsychiatric clinics.

A special individual record is prepared for each patient seen at a clinic. It contains all data on the diagnosis, treatment, and follow-up of the patient's condition, such as detailed anamnestic information, including data on family history, premorbid personality, social and living conditions, psychic traumata or other noxious factors immediately antecedent to or more remotely preceding the onset of the illness, and so on; the results of all clinical and paraclinical studies regarding the patient; epicrises from the hospitals where treatment was given; documents on the basis of which the patient has been assigned to work, pensioned, placed under guardianship, etc.; information on the treatment administered and its results, and much else.

The basic tasks assigned to the clinics are:

1. To study the prevalence and nature of psychiatric illness and its incidence in the country and the factors which play a role in the dynamics of these indices, i.e., to study the epidemiology of psychiatric diseases.

2. To ensure the early detection of psychiatric problems, their appropriate treatment (out of and in the hospital), and their active observation in the clinic.

3. To provide work, pensions, social and legal safeguards, welfare, and care for psychiatric patients.

4. To undertake prophylactic measures, particularly with regard to recurrent attacks, and to organize occupational therapy for patients with reduced working capacity.

5. To carry out health-education work among the people, in schools, in workers' collectives, on farms, etc.

The opportunities available to the psychiatric clinics for the study of mental illness and its incidence in general, as well as of some of its individual aspects, are very great. The clinics observe very large groups of patients over a long period and from a dynamic standpoint, since they are located throughout the entire country, with all its diverse conditions. Consequently, the results obtained are highly reliable. The clinics are in a much better position to study psychiatric illness and its incidence than are the hospitals and ordinary polyclinics. The psychiatric clinics can determine fully and most accurately the actual morbidity and incidence. Today we may state with reasonable certainty the overall psychiatric morbidity in Bulgaria, and also the morbidity in terms of individual nosologic entities. We have also been able to determine the changes in incidence for every recent year and for every disease.

Table I shows the psychiatric morbidity in absolute figures and per 1,000 inhabitants for the most important mental illnesses and as a whole, at the end of each year for the period 1952 to 1964.* It can be seen from this table that at the end of 1964 psychiatric morbidity in our country was 9.94 per 1,000 population. Moreover, it is immediately apparent that the following disorders rank first: oligophrenia, 3 per 1,000; epilepsy, 1.68 per 1,000; schizophrenia, 1.51 per 1,000. These are followed in order by neuroses, manic-depressive psychosis, etc.

The figures in Table 1 approximate those reported by some Soviet authors, who also studied the morbidity of the clinical method for relatively comparable diagnostic and nosologic categories.†

There is a notable constancy in the number of patients registered in different years, both in terms of morbidity as a whole and of individual nosologic categories. The number of clinic patients during four recent years increased from 1.12 to 1.14 per 1,000. If the increase in the population is taken, also, into account, then the rates are almost the same. If the morbidity rate is also of this order in the next three, five, or ten years, then the precise level of morbidity can be determined with great certainty. Hence it would be possible to draw very important theoretical and practical conclusions. It could, for example, be stated that the factors conducive to morbidity from mental illness are the same for different years and are not affected by random causes. From a practical standpoint, these regularities are important to the development of the psychiatric network (in and out

---

* The numerical data in this and the other tables were obtained in special investigations or from the annual reports of the neuropsychiatric clinics.

† It is worth noting that the extraordinary diversity of mental illnesses (as a whole or in terms of nosologic categories) is due to the fact, among others, that various criteria are used to make the psychiatric diagnosis, and the classifications employed are many and diverse. In this connection, we believe that a single set of international specifications for diagnosis and classification would contribute greatly to making it possible to compare the results obtained in different countries and would be extremely helpful in studying the epidemiology of mental illness. It would then be possible, too, to draw more definite conclusions about whether different geographic conditions, racial origin, living and cultural habits, types of diet, and other specific factors play a greater or smaller role in the dissemination of these disorders.

TABLE 1.

Psychiatric Morbidity in Absolute Figures and per 1,000 Inhabitants at the End of Each Year from 1952 to 1964.

Nosologic Entity	Year With Absolute Number and % of Population												
	1952	1953	1954	1955	1956	1957	1958	1959	1960	1961	1962	1963	1964
Schizophrenia	1,587 0.28	3,905 0.54	5,454 0.73	6,224 0.88	7,789 1.02	8,368 1.08	8,975 1.16	9,653 1.26	10,351 1.32	10,834 1.36	11,503 1.44	11,953 1.49	12,379 1.51
Epilepsy	618 0.09	2,456 0.33	4,551 0.61	6,673 0.89	8,458 1.11	9,551 1.22	10,246 1.32	11,245 1.44	11,764 1.50	12,534 1.58	13,427 1.68	13,985 1.75	14,466 1.68
Manic-Depressive Psychosis	356 0.05	797 0.11	1,088 0.15	1,375 0.18	1,663 0.22	1,966 0.24	2,128 0.27	2,427 0.31	2,603 0.33	2,764 0.35	2,971 0.37	3,072 0.38	3,371 0.41
Oligophrenia	800 0.11	3,175 0.43	5,687 0.76	8,134 1.08	10,909 1.44	12,340 1.66	13,910 1.79	15,807 2.03	17,246 2.19	18,924 2.38	20,987 2.62	22,676 2.83	24,560 3.00
Neuroses	1,082 0.15	2,669 0.31	4,816 0.64	4,424 0.58	4,863 0.64	4,915 0.64	5,357 0.69	4,907 0.63	4,926 0.63	4,571 0.58	4,751 0.59	3,798 0.47	3,698 0.45
Others	1,871 0.25	2,861 0.34	4,075 0.55	5,305 0.75	7,168 0.94	7,379 0.96	8,299 1.07	1,667 2.14	17,748 2.26	19,068 2.40	20,895 2.61	22,234 2.77	22,882 2.80
TOTAL	6,314 0.73	15,863 2.10	25,671 3.44	32,135 4.32	40,850 5.39	44,519 5.79	47,015 6.31	60,786 7.78	64,638 8.23	68,695 8.65	74,534 9.34	77,718 9.70	81,356 9.94

of the hospital), as well as to the determination of the need for medical personnel and drugs, and for the construction of psychiatric facilities.

In the case of some of the individual disorders, the constancy is even more pronounced. For example, in manic-depressive psychosis the morbidity ranges from 0.04 to 0.05 per 1,000 (with the sole exception of the year 1953, when it was 0.07 per 1,000). For some years, the number succumbing to this illness is virtually identical (1958, 305; 1959, 313; 1962, 326; 1957, 332).

With the data available on this illness today, it can be said with complete certainty that the causes which provoke it are extraordinarily constant, since in one fifteen-year period, almost exactly the same number of Bulgarians succumbed to this illness each year. If such facts are established in the statistics of other countries as well (with uniform diagnostic criteria), then the decisive role of endogenous factors in the origin of the disease can be definitely proclaimed, since the possible exogenous causes in the different countries show a wide variation.

To a significant degree, similar constancy is also manifested in morbidity from schizophrenia in Bulgaria. This has been clearly established in the last seven years, when, except for the years 1960 and 1961, morbidity varied within a range of 0.15–0.20 per 1,000.

Psychiatric clinics have also devoted a great deal of attention to the study of certain special problems in the epidemiology of psychiatric illnesses. Thus, for example, we now know how psychiatric illnesses are distributed in the different regions of the country and whether there is a tendency to seasonal manifestation of some illnesses.

We are still unable to say what causes the various morbidities in individual regions, but in the future, with more intensive study, we may discover some regular features. Interesting patterns emerge when comparing the frequency of illness in different groups of the population, such as between the urban and rural areas. I. Stoimenov and his coworkers found that morbidity from epilepsy and oligophrenia is observed significantly more frequently among the rural population than among the urban.[17, 18] Since investigation is likely to be better in an urban area, it is quite possible that there are definite regional factors contributing to the development of epilepsy and oligophrenia in the rural population. The authors reasoned that these factors stem from inferior living conditions in the rural areas; inadequate hygienic and dietary conditions during pregnancy; more frequent traumas during childbirth; and diseases in early childhood that result in damage to the nervous system.

Another interesting fact is that males incur these two disorders significantly more frequently than females. These data have been established in incontrovertible fashion for all regions of the country and for all age groups. The authors are not in a position to give a categorical explanation of these facts, but they think it highly probable that a certain role is played by the birth injuries which are considerably more frequent under the conditions of the rural lying-in home or in the domestic setting than in the large and well-equipped maternity homes in the cities. Birth injuries are more frequent and more severe in boys because their size at birth is greater than that of girls. Attention directed to these causes— if they are confirmed in the future by more convincing studies—could be of great practical importance in the prophylaxis of these disorders.

With respect to the age distribution of morbidity from epilepsy, it can be seen from the clinics' data that the number becoming ill in the first few years of life is greatest. It was established that 8.2 percent of all patients with epilepsy became ill in the first years of life; an average of 3 percent became ill in each year from the age of 2 to 4; 2 percent in each year in the period from 5 to 9 years; and 2.4 percent in the interval from 10 to 14 years. Of all patients with epilepsy, 73.3 percent manifested the illness before the age of 30.

At the present stage of the work of clinics, their attention is already being directed to more systematic investigations of the causes of mental illnesses. Although these studies are considerably more difficult, we believe that with the clinical method, based on exhaustive statistical studies, it will be possible to assemble a number of valuable facts of significance to the most difficult problem of psychiatry—the causes of psychiatric illnesses.

A particularly important problem for us, as for the world as a whole, is the study of schizophrenia. The data obtained by the clinics show that the frequency of this disease in Bulgaria is similar to the frequencies in other countries. The morbidity from schizophrenia in Bulgaria, at the end of 1964, was 1.51 per 1,000. The morbidity among females (according to data for 1959) was 1.31 per 1,000 and among males, 1.27 per 1,000. For every 100 men contracting the disease, 103 women succumb. If, however, a comparison is made of the morbidity among the rural and urban population, it is seen that for every 100 men in the urban population contracting the disease, 117.8 women succumb, and for the rural population, this ratio is 100:94.8. The overall morbidity among the urban population is 1.41 per 1,000, and among the rural population, 1.22 per 1,000.

In contrast to the polyclinics and hospitals, the neuropsychiatric clinics utilize a so-called "active method" for determining the mentally ill. The clinic physicians, together with their entire staff, and relying as well on the entire health network of the country (district health services in the countryside and cities, specialized establishments, schools, etc.), visit population centers and through examination procedures uncover psychiatric disorders. This approach is particularly concerned with the discovery of oligophrenia, epilepsy, psychopathies, and neuroses, which are not always so conspicuous in their manifestations as to cause relatives to take patients to the clinics for study and treatment. Much cooperation in this tracing activity is afforded the neuropsychiatric clinics by the social organizations, and especially by the health commissions of the Red Cross, Fatherland Front, etc.

It must also be noted that in the fifteen years of their life, the clinics have made themselves quite popular among the population, having duly clarified their medical and social role in all mental illness. If it is borne in mind that all examinations and all the services rendered to the mentally ill (as well as all medical assistance in general) in Bulgaria are completely free of charge, it becomes clear why there is no serious interference with the early detection and timely treatment of the mentally ill.

The indices for the early detection of disease are being revised constantly according to the data of the neuropsychiatric clinics. Thus, for example, in 1962, 7.2 percent of the patients were admitted to the clinic as early as the first month of their illness (the data apply to the country as a whole), and in 1964, this percentage was 12.40. In some of the clinics, this index is significantly higher (for example, in the regional neuropsychiatric clinic in Sofia, 17.2 percent of all patients were admitted to the clinic as early as the first month). As far as individual disorders are concerned, some of the clinics record very good results. The regional neuropsychiatric clinic at Plovdiv treated 28.8 percent of the schizophrenic patients in the clinic and the Russe clinic, 44.9 percent.[13]

Though great difficulties are still encountered in the initial detection of the mentally ill, the clinics are very active in their follow-up of patients, which is of exceptional importance for the prophylaxis of recurrent attacks of the illness and for the social situation of the patients. Once the patient has been admitted to a neuropsychiatric clinic, he is called in regularly thereafter for follow-up examinations, or he is visited in his home by a district psychiatrist.

Each clinic has at its disposal, as well as its own beds in the inpatient unit of the clinic, the beds in a corresponding psychiatric hospital. A special advantage of the Bulgarian psychiatric organization is the interaction of these two basic institutions, the neuropsychiatric clinic and the psychiatric hospital. Immediately after the existence of a psychiatric disorder has been established, the clinic sends the patient to the regional hospital (if it deems this necessary), with all pertinent anamnestic and other studies accomplished at the clinic. The psychiatric hospital may ask the clinic for supplementary information of a social or similar nature, needed for complete elucidation of the case.

The need for hospital treatment in a psychiatric hospital is decided by the clinic physician. The hospital physicians, however, also determine whether the patient requires hospitalization. In the case of a dispute as to whether or not to admit, joint consultation between the clinic and regional hospital provides the answer.

The mentally ill in Bulgaria can be admitted without special authorization from the office of the district attorney or a court. Only when the patient or his family refuse hospitalization and the patient represents a danger to those around him, is the matter settled by a decision of the district attorney's office. In such cases, the court, after forensic psychiatric testimony, decrees or rejects compulsory treatment in a psychiatric hospital. The length of treatment is usually not determined in advance but is left up to the physicians administering the treatment. These physicians also decide when the treatment has been completed, at which time they present their conclusion in writing to the court. The court has the sole right to cancel compulsory treatment.

On completion of treatment in the hospital, and in conjunction with the patient's discharge, a detailed epicrisis of the examination, treatment and diagnosis is dispatched to the clinic. Also required at this time are recommendations to the clinic with respect to further treatment, work, and any other matters relating to the health and social situation of the patient. Thus, immediately after the patient goes home, the clinic is fully informed of his condition and of the hospital's recommendations, as well as of whatever else it deems necessary for the further care of the patient.

Today, in an era of widespread application of neuroloptics in the treatment of psychiatric disorders, the role and significance of the neuropsychiatric clinics is increasing considerably, since for a large proportion of patients aftercare treatment with neuroloptics is administered at home. The condition of the mentally ill and the administration of this treatment cannot be monitored in establishments that do not have special facilities for active clinical observation. The neuropsychiatric clinics are equipped for this important task, since they have the financial resources for the free administration of drugs to the patients. The clinics are equipped with laboratories which, in addition to the studies required for diagnosis and treatment, make tests of whether patients are taking the prescribed drugs at home.

The volume of the clinics' work can be judged, in part, from the number of examinations made. The number of ambulatory patients examined in 1964 was 194,486; of these 22,424 (or 11.5 percent) of the examinations were carried out in the patients' homes. The number of examinations for each patient depends on the group to which he belongs (nature of illness, stage of disease, need for support therapy, etc.) and ranges from 1 to 3.8 examinations per patient per year. Psychiatric inpatient establishments whose prophylactic efforts are largely therapy-oriented are not in a position to conduct such a large number of psychiatric examinations, and neither are establishments of the general health network that have no special orientation toward the mentally ill. Through the clinics, the outpatient organization of psychiatric treatment is coming into increasingly close contact with the population. A good index of this is the constantly increasing number of examinations, and particularly of visits to the patients' homes.

Eighty-two clinic psychiatrists, plus eight other psychiatrists in the clinic sections of psychiatric hospitals and psychiatric consulting rooms at hospitals for somatic diseases or ninety physicians in all, provide clinic treatment for the approximately 8,200,000 persons in Bulgaria (1965). This means that the patient load of each physician in the clinic network is about 89,000.* In the next three to five years, the number of physicians will increase so that the patient load of each physician will be approximately 60,000. Working in the neuropsychiatric clinics, in addition to the psychiatrists, are nurses (with a secondary medical education), who also make calls at the patients' homes, inquire as to their condition, and report all their observations to the doctors. With this staff, the neuropsychiatric clinics, in addition to their clinic activity also carry out therapeutic activity in the inpatient units which have 470 beds in the entire country.

---

* If the number of psychiatrists in the psychiatric hospitals is also taken into account, then the patient load in Bulgaria is 35,000 per psychiatrist. In the psychiatric clinics, hospitals, and rest homes there are 141 psychiatrists at work; of these, 33 are scientific workers and teachers. In the country as a whole, the number of psychiatrists at the end of 1964 was 231.

JOBS, TRUSTS, WELFARE, AND
LEGAL PROTECTION FOR THE MENTALLY ILL

The clinics look after the jobs of the patients whenever this is necessary. They see to it that patients are provided with good working conditions and a short working day. In planning a patient's work program, the clinic can make use of the following approaches: (a) shifting the patient to work in the same or another enterprise better suited to his disorder than his regular employment. The pay is not reduced on this transfer to easier work. A work program of this sort lasts for a specified term (three, six, or twelve months), after which the patient is reexamined to determine whether the work program should be continued or not; (b) granting sick leave with pay for a limited period; (c) in the case of an unfavorable course of the disease, offering the sick worker a pension for a period of one or two years, after which he is reexamined, and, depending on his condition, either the term of the pension is extended or he goes back to work.

The clinics undertake the social and legal protection of the mentally ill, utilizing the trust system for the protection of the property and rights of the mentally ill, etc. According to S. Bachev and T. Stankushev,[12, 14] in 1961, 12.4 percent of all clinic-treated patients over the age of eighteen years required supervision, and 11 percent of these, mainly at the initiative of the clinics, were placed under wardship. The largest percentage of patients who required supervision were those with traumatic damage to the central nervous system, senile psychoses, atherosclerosis, oligophrenia, serious schizophrenia, and epileptic personality change.

When it becomes necessary to make the patient a ward, the clinic's opinion is usually accepted on this point, and especially that of the regional psychiatrist. The clinic itself has the right to require the placement of certain patients under wardship.

In the clinic context, a forensic psychiatric report is most frequently accomplished in the following way: The court needs an expert's report, in most instances from the clinic, since the commission which prepares the report usually includes a legal psychiatrist in addition to the regional psychiatrist, who is most familiar with the patient's condition before the commission of the illegal act. When hospital observation is ordered because of the commission of an act dangerous to the public, the physicians investigating and treating the patient participate in the formulation of the expert's report. Patients stay for forensic psychiatric certification in psychiatric inpatient units. Those patients for whom strict confinement is necessary stay in special forensic-psychiatry sections at the psychiatric clinic of the Faculty of Medicine in Sofia, at the Scientific Research Institute of Neurology and Psychiatry in Sofia, or at the psychiatric hospital in Lovech.

MENTAL HYGIENE AND PSYCHOPROPHYLACTIC MEASURES

The social welfare work of the clinics is of exceptionally great significance, since through it the clinic becomes thoroughly acquainted with the patient's family and living conditions. The clinic's regional psychiatrist also provides aid and collaboration, when needed, to the patient's family to improve the patient's living conditions. Moreover, the clinic psychiatrist gives regular advice to the family on how to care for the patient and how best to arrange and protect his interests as a patient.

Because the causes of the most important mental illnesses are unknown, it is difficult—indeed, almost impossible—to adopt a purposeful approach to the prevention of mental illnesses prior to the first attack. Of course, measures to prevent recurrent attacks are very important. The clinics, because of their dynamic observation of the mentally ill, can often prolong remissions and space out recurrences. They do not passively await the onset of the next attack in order to treat it but make serious efforts to delay attacks through treatment with psychopharmacologic agents. For example, it is the prevailing opinion in Bulgaria that pharmacologic prophylaxis is of the greatest importance in schizophrenia.

The clinics have organized workshops for patients who are out of work because of their illness. These occupational-therapy outpatient units and workshops take in a considerable number of patients from the cities. Their time outside working hours is spent at home. During their working time, facilities are afforded them for rest (on the day-hospital principle), and food and various diversions are provided. For the work performed, the patients receive monetary compensation. Thus, not only is a good rehabilitation program provided for the patients, but also, through a system of duly apportioned work and diversion, a prophylactic influence is exerted even on so-called endogenous psychoses.

The neuropsychiatric clinics organize and undertake prophylactic examinations on their own or in collaboration with other therapeutic and prophylactic establishments, at businesses in which there is a risk of the development of various mental disorders. Such examinations are most frequent in textile plants and factories, where the workers often risk damage to the nervous system (intoxication, noise, dust, etc.). Where illness threatens, it is suggested to management that it institute prophylactic measures and send persons who have become ill for treatment.

One special type of activity which is carried on extensively by the clinics, and which has proved to be exceptionally beneficial, is the treatment of neurotic speech disorders (stammering). The clinics, with the help of the school physicians and teachers, seek out stammerers and treat them. The patients either go to the outpatient unit of the clinic from two to four times a week in groups of three, five or eight persons, or else enter the inpatient unit, where in the course of thirty to sixty days systematic treatment is carried out. A very successful approach utilized by the clinics is the organization of summer camps for children, where a special program of courses of this type are given in a restful setting. There are already quite well-trained psychiatry specialists in Bulgaria who are engaged in devising various methods for the treatment of neurotic speech disorders on a scientific basis.

HEALTH EDUCATION

The clinics do an enormous amount of work in health education among the population. They deal mainly with matters directly or indirectly related to mental hygiene and the psychoprophylaxis of mental disorders; hygiene of intellectual and physical work; the problems of alcoholism; the problems of fitness, etc. Hundreds of talks are given by the clinics' physicians before plant and office groups, etc., where a series of questions about the nature of mental illnesses is explained in plain terms. The main emphasis is on prophylaxis and the opportunities for timely treatment and special attention is paid to the iatrogenic factor and ways of avoiding it.

Such talks are also delivered to the patients in the inpatient units and to former patients who have kept up their contact with the clinics after their recovery. In addition, various forms of radio broadcasting, meetings, and visual aids are utilized. Recently, there has been more purposeful scrutiny of the problems of alcoholism and tobacco smoking and of the problems and treatment of neuroses. Also the causes and prevention of oligophrenia are being studied in conjunction with specialists in other medical fields (obstetricians, pediatricians; specialists in infectious diseases, etc.)

PSYCHIATRIC TREATMENT IN HOSPITALS

Hospital psychiatric treatment in Bulgaria is available through the following establishments:

1. Psychiatric clinics at all educational and scientific research establishments;

   a Psychiatric clinic of the Faculty of Medicine in Sofia,

   b Psychiatric clinic of the Scientific Research Institute of Neurology and Psychiatry in Sofia,

   c Psychiatric clinic of the Institute for the Postgraduate Training and Specialization of Physicians (at the Scientific Research Institute of Neurology and Psychiatry), Sofia,

   d Psychiatric clinic of the Faculty of Medicine in Plovdiv,

   e Psychiatric clinic of the Faculty of Medicine in Varna.

In all, then, there are 355 beds in the five psychiatric clinics.

2. Psychiatric hospitals (ten in number) with a total of 2,084 beds.

3. Inpatient units of the neuropsychiatric dispensaries, with a total of 470 beds.

4. Psychiatric centers, with a total of 360 beds.

Altogether there are 3,269 beds in the inpatient psychiatric establishments of Bulgaria.

In addition to these, there are 3,208 beds in the special homes for social care (2,164 for adults with mental defects, and 1,044 for children with mental defects). Lodged in this type of establishment are patients whose mental disorder is permanent—most frequently those suffering from oligophrenia (idiots and imbeciles), severe epileptic deterioration, and severe traumatic dementia.

In Bulgaria, then, there are 6,477 beds for the hospitalization of the mentally ill, or 0.81 beds per 1,000 population.

With this supply of beds, there is of course overcrowding of the psychiatric establishments, as in almost all countries. Thus, for example, according to Stoimenov's data, there were 10 percent more patients in the country's inpatient establishments in 1960 than there were beds.

The plan for the development of the hospital network envisages 1.5 beds per 1,000 population by the year 1980. This figure will be far below the figures attained in some countries, but it is estimated that this

TABLE 2.

Number and Percentage of Patients Treated, according to Diagnosis.

Diagnosis	Treated		Untreated		Total Hospitalized Patients
	Number	%	Number	%	
Schizophrenia	1,100	59.2	760	40.8	1,860
Epilepsy	190	82.7	40	17.3	230
Manic-Depressive Psychosis	130	92.8	10	7.2	140
Oligophrenia	70	36.8	110	63.2	180
Other	490	79.5	160	24.5	650
TOTAL	1,980	64.6	1,080	35.4	3,060
Number of these exhibiting chronic symptoms	1,010	51.3	960	48.7	1,950

number of beds will meet the needs for hospital treatment. We consider that the presence of the neuropsychiatric clinics in Bulgaria relieves the psychiatric hospitals to a significant extent, and although with fewer beds, helps to meet the great need for psychiatric treatment. Since prolonged hospitalization is not always necessary for all patients, and since they are allowed to stay in their usual domestic and social environment when their condition so permits under the uninterrupted care of the neuropsychiatric clinics, the need for psychiatric hospital treatment will be met to an adequate degree by this number of beds.

An important index of the work of the hospital establishments is the number of patients treated. Ten to fifteen years ago, the majority of the patients were not treated, owing to the chronic nature of their illness. Table 2 shows the number of patients treated and their distribution according to diagnosis in the inpatient establishments in 1961. Today, these indices are even higher, since the application of neuroleptics is more widespread.

PROBLEMS CONFRONTING THE
PSYCHIATRIC HOSPITAL NETWORK

It seems to us that the most important problem is the constant increase in the number of chronically ill and elderly patients. This phenomenon is observed in all the countries of the world. Its explanation in Bulgaria is that an ever greater proportion of the mentally ill—thanks to active treatment of their somatic illnesses and good general care and feeding—reach quite an advanced age. Another cause is the increasing average lifespan of the population in our country. Thus, for example, in 1964, the average lifespan for women was seventy-one years, and for men, sixty-eight years—which, in turn, increases the number of senile psychoses.

It is probable in view of these findings that Sjogren and Larsen point out that, with increasing age, the risk of developing a mental illness also increases. We do not wholly share this view, since in the case of some illnesses, the risk of morbidity decreases with increasing age (e.g., epilepsy, schizophrenia, manic-depressive psychosis, and oligophrenia). The increase in morbidity which is directly proportional to age, applies mostly to senile and presenile psychoses.

The number and percentage of patients in our psychiatric establishments, in terms of age distribution, can be seen from Table 3. This table offers a basis for the following conclusions: (a) the diagnosis encountered

TABLE 3.

Distribution of Patients in Inpatient Establishments according to Diagnosis, Age and Sex in 1961 (I. Stoimenov and coworkers).*

Diagnosis	Age and Sex																TOTAL	
	10–19		20–29		30–39		40–49		50–59		60–69		Over 70		Total		Number	%
	M	F	M	F	M	F	M	F	M	F	M	F	M	F	M	F		
Schizophrenia	30	40	170	100	450	380	220	170	70	160	50	20			990	870	1,860	61.0
Epilepsy	20		20	40	50		30	20	30	20					150	80	230	7.5
Manic-Depressive Psychosis	10		10		30			20	20	30	10	10			80	60	140	4.6
Oligophrenia	20		60	30	10	10		10	30		10				130	50	180	5.5
Other	10		50	60	60	30	100	60	110	80	10	30	20	30	360	290	650	21.4
TOTAL	90	40	310	230	600	420	350	280	260	290	80	60	20	30	1,710	1,350	3,060	100.0

* The figures are rounded off to ten, since the study was done on a 10 percent sample of the number of all patients.

TABLE 4.

Number and Percentage of Patients Registered in the Neuropsychiatric Clinics
and Undergoing Treatment in the Inpatient Establishments in
1961 (I. Stoimenov and coworkers).

Diagnosis	Registered in Clinics		Hospitalized		% of All Clinic Patients in Hospitals
	Number	%	Number	%	
Schizophrenia	9,653	15.9	1,860	61	19.3
Epilepsy	11,245	18.5	230	7.5	2.4
Manic-Depressive Psychosis	2,427	4.0	140	4.6	5.8
Oligophrenia	15,807	26.1	180	5.5	1.1
Other	21,604	35.5	650	21.4	4.4
TOTAL	60,736	100.0	3,060	100.0	5.1

most frequently in our psychiatric establishments is schizophrenia (62 percent); (b) the largest number of patients undergoing treatment are aged 30–39 years (30 percent of all patients), followed by those aged 40–49 years (20 percent).

It is interesting to compare the number undergoing treatment with the number of registered mental patients. This is shown on Table 4. It is apparent from this table that schizophrenia accounts for only 15.9% of the patients registered in the clinics and that schizophrenics take up 61% of the beds in inpatient establishments. Of the patients with schizophrenia, 19.3% are cared for in the inpatient establishments, followed, far behind, by those with epilepsy (2.4%).

Table 5 shows the distribution of patients in terms of the length of their hospitalization. It is evident that about 38% (1,160 patients) have been hospitalized for more than a year, and 24.5% (750 patients) for more than three years. This is eloquent testimony to the choking of the hospital establishments with chronically ill patients. More than 64% of the patients undergoing treatment exhibit chronic illness, and only 35% are patients with acute illness.

Another serious problem is the lack of geriatrically oriented hospital establishments. As of today, only a beginning has been made, with the organization of a center for geriatrics (at the Ministry of National Health), which is concerned with geriatric psychiatry.

An important problem for Bulgarian psychiatry is the organization of occupational therapy. Despite what has been achieved in the last one or two decades, there is still a large proportion of patients who are not engaged in work activity. Occupational therapy is not diversified enough and is not suitable for the patients' conditions in all cases. One of the objective reasons for this is the existence of hospital establishments with few beds. There is also a lack of cultural and diversion therapy, due mainly to the shortage of well-trained personnel in this field.

The staff-patient ratio in the hospital establishments is good. Thus, for the total of 3,269 beds there are 126 physicians, or 26 beds to each psychiatrist.

In their general appearance, the psychiatric hospitals and clinics are coming more and more to resemble the establishments for general somatic diseases. They have all the necessary laboratories and equipment for complete investigation of the status of the patients' health. Modern facilities for treatment are available. The state provides adequate means—free of charge—for the complex treatment of all mental patients.

TABLE 5.

Distribution of Patients in Inpatient Establishments according to Duration of Hospitalization and Diagnosis (1961).

Diagnosis	Period of Hospitalization									
	Up to 3 mo.	4–6 mo.	7–12 mo.	1–2 yr.	2–3 yr.	3–5 yr.	6–10 yr.	11 yr. or more	not indicated	TOTAL
Schizophrenia	510	200	200	120	170	380	180	70	30	1,860
Epilepsy	90	10	50	30		30	10	10		230
Manic-Depressive Psychosis	120	10				10				140
Oligophrenia	50	30	20	20	20	10	20		10	180
Other	440	30	80	40	20	20		10	10	650
TOTAL	1,210	280	350	210	210	450	210	90	50	3,060
Number of these exhibiting chronic symptoms	380	140	270	200	200	440	210	90	40	1,970

POSTGRADUATE TRAINING IN PSYCHIATRY

As of today, only two specialties in psychiatry have been approved in the regulations on specialties in Bulgaria: General Psychiatry and Child Psychiatry. The latter specialty is obtained after the specialty in General Psychiatry has already been taken and a probationary period in the field of child psychiatry of at least three years has been completed.

The minor specialties that existed before 1965—in Forensic Psychiatry and in the Labor Expertise of Mental Illnesses—have been deleted from the nomenclature, since the need for them today is very limited. However, a more important consideration which led the Council on Teaching Methodology of the Ministry of National Health and Social Welfare to do away with these specialties was the understanding that any well-trained clinical psychiatrist can cope successfully with the scientific and practical exigencies of forensic psychiatric expertise. The opinion prevailed that many narrow specialties in psychiatry would impede the integral development of physician-psychiatrists. The psychiatrist's ability to deal with the problems of forensic psychiatry, labor expertise, and organizational matters must be an aspect of the specialty of General Psychiatry that will not fully engage his attention.

According to the regulations for obtaining specialty status in Bulgaria, any physician who has had at least three years of therapeutic and diagnostic work in a univeristy psychiatric clinic or hospital directed by a specialist psychiatrist has the right to present himself for acquisition of specialist status before a commission of the Ministry of National Health, which is made up of professors and eminent specialists.

Since 1950, a higher-educational establishment has existed in Bulgaria, which has as its basic purpose the handling of questions relating to the specialization and postgraduate training of physicians. It is directed by the Institute for the Specialization and Postgraduate Training of Physicians (ISUL) and has a considerable number of departments. The Department of Psychiatry is directed by Professor E. Sharankov. The basic task of this department in the field of specialization is to organize various courses in psychiatry, in which physicians after having worked for several years in the provincial or district clinics, perfect their knowledge through systematic theoretical and practical work.

For fifteen years now, the Department of Psychiatry of the ISUL has organized a large number of courses lasting twelve, nine or six months.

Through its lecture rooms have passed almost all today's young Bulgarian specialists in psychiatry. Many of them become directors of clinics, hospitals or psychiatric consulting rooms after studying at the ISUL.

Another form of specialist training in psychiatry—in our opinion, the best in terms of quality—is the so-called clinical internship. This involves the securing, by competition, of a state post as a clinical intern by a young physician who has completed his obligatory three-year rural-probation period. As well as performing practical work, the clinical intern takes a series of examinations in psychology, general psychiatry, and special psychiatry. He works for six months in a neurological clinic and is then examined in neurology. At the end of his three-year period, the candidate presents himself before the Ministry of National Health for an examination leading to a specialty in psychiatry. Many good specialists are thus trained, and they are generally appointed section chiefs in psychiatric hospitals in the provinces.

A very interesting and important matter is that of the continuous qualification of Bulgarian physicians. The basic responsibility for this continued postgraduate training of specialists in Bulgaria is also assigned to the ISUL. Of course, the postgraduate training of physicians is also accomplished in a number of other highly specialized clinics and departments, but the largest share of this work, as well as its methodological direction, is the responsibility of the ISUL. The Department of Psychiatry of the ISUL has carried on very extensive activity in the postgraduate training of psychiatrists for fifteen years now. In the theoretical and practical courses organized by the ISUL, lectures are delivered by professors and eminent specialists. Over a period of one to four months, these courses for postgraduate training take up narrow and, at the same time, important problems in psychiatry, for example, current problems of forensic psychiatry, new trends in clinic work, problems of psychotherapy, aspects of pharmacologic treatment and psychotherapy, and the treatment of neurotic speech disorders.

In 1966, the Department of Psychiatry of the ISUL offered several new courses for the postgraduate training of specialists, viz., the clinical aspects and therapy of exogenous psychoses (one month), problems of geriatic psychiatry (two months), and the psychology of work for neurologists, psychiatrists, and psychologists from the medical first-aid sections of the large enterprises.

A higher form of scientific postgraduate training is the so-called "aspiranture" (research postgraduate). One secures a state post as an "aspirant" or obtains, by competition, the right to defend a scientific monograph. Many young psychiatrists, including some from the outlying areas, have successfully prepared and defended dissertations before the faculties of higher educational establishments and the Institute of Neurology and Psychiatry (which has the right to direct and award scientific degrees) and have obtained the degree of Candidate in Medical Sciences. Over and above the public recognition of the author's scientific achievements, this degree entails a considerable salary raise for its holder (thirty levs* for a candidate in medical sciences, fifty levs for a Doctor of Medical Sciences).

Thanks to the systematic concern of the state for the postgraduate training of Bulgarian physicians, the number of specialists in psychiatry is steadily increasing. During the time in which their continuing qualification is kept up to date through periodic courses, the specialists not only receive their full salary but also get additional compensation for expenses incurred during the period of their specialization or postgraduate training.

The special training of secondary medical workers is carried out in the hospitals themselves. In Bulgaria today, special schools for psychiatric nurses are lacking. Secondary medical education is the same for all nurses —a three-year course after graduation from the "gymnasium" (junior-college-level preparatory school). It would be better, however, to set up schools at the large psychiatric hospitals, and consideration is now being given to this idea in Bulgaria.

The training of occupational therapists, cultural therapists, and other auxiliary personnel takes place separately. In these fields, too, a broader education is necessary, since personnel of this type are of great importance in conducting an up-to-date therapeutic and rehabilitation program.

THE PLACE OF PSYCHIATRY IN THE SYSTEM OF MEDICAL EDUCATION

The psychiatry course is included in the fifth year of medical education. The sixth year is designed solely for the clinical training of the students, and only ten days are set aside for practical work in psychiatry.

The schedule for the lecture course in psychiatry comprises a total of seventy-five hours, of which forty-five hours are devoted to lectures and

* 1.17 leva = U.S. $1.

thirty hours to practical exercises. It is concentrated in one semester. It must be pointed out that this small number of lecture hours is completely inadequate for thorough teaching of the material stipulated in the program. Attempts to increase the number of hours spent on psychiatry meet with opposition on the part of the faculty councils since the weekly study load of the students (lectures and exercises) must not exceed thirty-two hours.

Psychiatry occupies an important position in the system of higher medical education. This is true not only because it explains a number of interesting illnesses of real practical importance but also because it prepares the students to develop a good understanding of the human psyche, to be able to form proper relationships with patients, and—most important —to apply effectively the most universal method of treatment in medicine psychotherapy.

The curriculum itself consists of two parts: Included in the first part are problems of general psychopathology, presented as a propadeutic course; in the second part clinical psychiatry is studied and the most important nosologic entities and their treatments are studied. All lectures involve clinical demonstrations, educational films, tables, diagrams, and tape recordings, which exert a complex effect on the listeners and contribute to a more complete assimilation of the teaching material.

The practical exercises are conducted at the bedside of the patients. Each student must master the methods of clinical investigation of mental patients, including examination of cerebrospinal fluid, EEG, whatever else is relevant to the psychosomatic status and health of a patient. Each group of students consists of six to ten persons and is under the direct guidance of an assistant, who teaches them by practical demonstration and is responsible for their individual training.

Important in the practical education of Bulgarian psychiatrists is the probationary period, which, as pointed out, occurs in the sixth year of medical school. Although it is brief, through it the probationers are able to consider anew, in concise fashion but at a higher level, the nosologic entities most important for practice, such as the neuroses, oligophrenia, symptomatic psychoses, schizophrenia, and epilepsy, from both a clinical and a therapeutic standpoint. Particular attention is paid to psychopharmacologic therapy. The knowledge the students acquire about the therapeutic virtues of the various types of psychotherapeutic substances are also needed by them in the formulation of therapeutic programs, in mental, as well as in somatic illnesses.

It is essential to point out that, since 1964, the curriculum for medical education has included an optional course on medical psychology. As of today, the lectures are given by the Department of Psychiatry of the Faculties of Medicine in Sofia, Plovidiv, and Varna, since there are still not enough qualified teachers of medical psychology in Bulgaria.

Unlike a number of Western and Eastern schools, Bulgarian medical departments believe that medical psychology in the system of higher medical education should not repeat the problems of general psychopathology or give the essence of general psychology. We are of the opinion that a program of medical psychology should be considered an applied psychology of medicine. It should include problems peculiar to the mentality of people with somatic illnesses, the psychological relationship between doctor and patient, the most common psychological problems in the organization of the hospital regime, and the basic psychological premises of psychotherapy, mental hygiene, psychoprophylaxis, etc. Of great importance also are the practical problems considered above, such as rehabilitation, work programs, and pensioning for illness.

The authors' two years' experience in the teaching of medical psychiatry in Bulgaria has demonstrated to them the exceptionally great importance of this discipline for the formation of correct relationships between a doctor and his patients and their relatives, and its importance, too, in shaping his view of life and his education as a physician-humanist. The course in medical psychology is attended not only by medical students but also by students of psychology, pedagogy, the training of defectives, and others. Thus, this discipline has great importance in the education of a number of specialists.

We must call attention to the so-called "student autonomous scientific activity." As in all other departments, circles consisting each of about ten or twelve students have been formed in the department of psychiatry. Besides preparing for clinical practice, the members of these circles work up scientific problems of a clinical-statistical or clinical-experimental nature. All student science circles are directed by a qualified teacher. Some students from psychiatry circles have participated successfully in scientific symposia at local or national conferences on student science activity. The best of these works are published in the student science journal, *Praemedicus*.

Twelve years of experience with student psychiatry circles have shown that the members of these clubs are the most suitable personnel for scientific and practical work in the field of psychiatry after they receive their medical dipolmas. When they start to work in the psychiatric network, they are prepared to cope immediately with current diagnostic and therapeutic problems—something which other young physicians who did not join the circles and lack special preliminary preparation are not in a position to do.

In closing our account of the development, current status, and prospects of Bulgarian psychiatry, we should take note of certain social gains which have been acquired from the state by the personnel working in psychiatric establishments.

The work of physicians, graduate nurses, occupational therapists, etc., in the neuropsychiatric clinics is considered to be a risk to health. Because of this, the working time of the personnel has been reduced to thirty-five hours a week, as against forty-five hours for establishments concerned with somatic health. The workers in the psychiatric-health network get a twelve-day extension of the normal annual holiday and a higher monthly pay. Proposals have been prepared that will ensure more favorable conditions for the pensioning of these personnel.

These social gains for workers in the psychiatric establishments have helped considerably to attract better personnel to psychiatry (mostly nurses and orderlies), of whom a certain lack is still felt in other branches of medical practice.

References

1. S. DOBREVA, V. IONCHEV, S. VLAEV, AND K. TSAFAROV: Neuropsychiatric Treatment of Children and Adolescents—Tasks and Prospects, *Bulletin of the Scientific Research Institute of Neurology and Psychiatry*, 8 (1):5–8 (1964).

2. TS. KRISTANOV: "Natural Science in Medieval Bulgaria," Bulgarian Academy of Sciences, Sofia, 1954.

3. N. KRUSTNIKOV: "The Therapeutic Effect of Artificially Provoked Reproduction of Pathogenic Experiences," 1929.

4. G. LOZANOV AND A. ATANASOV: Psychotherapy and Cultural Therapy in the Neuropsychiatric Clinics, *Bulletin of the Scientific Research Institute of Neurology and Psychiatry*, 8 (1):22–35 (1964).

5. ZH. MOLKHOV: On Some Problems of Mental Health and Psychiatric Treatment of Old People, *Neurology, Psychiatry and Neurosurgery*, 3 (1):1–7 (1964).

6. ZH. MOLKHOV, A. SIRAKOV, AND M. TSVETKOVA: Ten Years of Outpatient Psychiatric Treatment, *Bulletin of the Scientific Research Institute of Neurology and Psychiatry*, 8 (1):32–35 (1964).

7. ZH. MOLKHOV, M. TSVETKOVA, S. VACHEV, AND T. STANKUSHEV: On Certain Problems of Newly Recorded Illness During 1961, *Transactions of the Scientific Research Institute of Neurology and Psychiatry*, 10:101–106 (1964).

8. G. NASTEV, ZH. MOLKHOV, AND I. TEMKOV: Status and Tasks of Neuropsychiatric Treatment in This Country, *Scientific Transactions of the NIIHP*, 1:55–81 (1953/54).

9. D. PANTELEEV, A. KURSHUTSKI, AND L. MILUSHEV: Occupational Therapy and Therapeutic Physical Culture in the Outpatient Rehabilitation of Mental Patients, *Bulletin of the Scientific Research Institute of Neurology and Psychiatry*, 8 (1):9–12 (1964).

10. E. SHARANKOV, M. TSVETKOVA, AND S. SHIVACHEVA: The Contemporary Prophylaxis of Mental Illnesses in This Country, *Bulletin of the Scientific Research Institute of Neurology and Psychiatry*, 8 (1):1–4 (1964).

11. A. SIRAKOV, R. RASHEV, AND M. TSVETKOVA: Epilepsy in Bulgaria, *Modern Medicine*, 9 (10):33–41 (1958).

12. T. STANKUSHEV AND P. DONCHEV: Some Current Problems in the Organization of Outpatient Forensic Psychiatric Treatment, *Bulletin of the Scientific Research Institute of Neurology and Psychiatry*, 8 (1):17–21 (1964).

13. T. STANKUSHEV AND R. IVANOV: The Problem of the Early Clinic Treatment of the Mentally Ill, *Bulletin of the Scientific Research Institute of Neurology and Psychiatry*, 8 (1):37–38 (1964).

14. I. STOIMENOV, A. SIRAKOV, AND S. BACHEV: The Necessity of Expanding and Decentralizing Outpatient Psychiatric Treatment, *Bulletin*

of the Scientific Research Institute of Neurology and Psychiatry, 8 (1):39–43 (1964).

15. I. STOIMENOV, S. DOBREVA, S. BACHEV, AND M. KOICHEVA: Breakdown of Patients Undergoing Treatment of Psychiatric Establishments, *Bulletin of the Scientific Research Institute of Neurology and Psychiatry* 5(3/4):78–84 (1961).

16. I. STOIMENOV, A. SIRAKOV, S. BACHEV, AND M. KOICHEVA: Volume and Nature of Psychiatric Morbidity and Its Incidence in Bulgaria, *Neurology, Psychiatry and Neurosurgery*, 3 (1):7–16 (1964).

17. I. TEMKOV: Development of Bulgarian Psychiatric Science in Neuropsychiatric Treatment, S. S. *Korsakov Journal of Neuropathology and Psychiatry*, 57 (1):114–123 (1957).

18. I. TEMKOV: Development of Psychiatry in Bulgaria, *Neurology, Psychiatry and Neurosurgery* 3 (4):245–249 (1964).

19. I. TEMKOV AND S. IZRAEL: The First Woman Physician, the First Woman Psychiatrist in This Country, *Bulletin of the Scientific Research Institute of Neurology and Psychiatry*, 2 (1):46–47 (1958).

20. I. TEMKOV: On the Basic Methodologic Problems of Neurology and Psychiatry, *Health Front*, (16, 17, 23, 24, 25, 26, 27) (1950).

21. I. TEMKOV: Stefan Danadzhiev—Founder of Bulgarian Psychiatry, *Modern Medicine*, 9 (10):143–151 (1958).

22. I. TEMKOV, KH. DIMITROV, AND M. GULUBOVA: Nikola Gavrilov Krustnikov—Eminent Bulgarian Psychiatrist, *Modern Medicine*, 7(1): 109–119 (1956).

23. I. TEMKOV, V. IVANOV, AND KH. KHRISTOZOV: Development of Bulgarian Psychiatric Science, *Scientific Transactions of the NIINP*, 1:3–36 (1953/54).

24. M. TSVETKOVA, ZH. MOLKHOV, AND I. LIUBENOVA: Contribution to the Problem of Psychiatric Hospital Construction in This Country, *Neurology and Psychiatry*, 2 (2):60–70 (1963).

25. M. TSVETKOVA, TS. TIKHOLOV, AND B. CHAKMAKOV: Problems of Labor Expertise and the Work Programs of the Mentally Ill in Outpatient Treatment, *Bulletin of the Scientific Research Institute of Neurology and Psychiatry*, 8 (1):13–16 (1964).

26. G. UZUNOV: On Some Social Problems of Psychiatry in This Country, *Modern Medicine*, 12 (6):3–17 (1961).

27. G. UZUNOV, S. DOBREVA, ZH. MOLKHOV, AND T. STANKUSHKEV: Outpatient Psychiatric Treatment in this Country—Status, Tasks and Perspectives for Development, *Neurology, Psychiatry, and Neurosurgery*, 3 (2):65–82 (1964).

28. G. UZUNOV AND A. SIRAKOV: Status of Neuropsychiatric Treatment in Bulgaria—Prospects for Its Growth, *Modern Medicine*, 11 (7/8):191–202 (1960).

CHAPTER NINE

Some Aspects of Rumanian Psychiatry

BY

DR. A. DOSIES, DR. CONSTANTA PARHON-
STEFANESCU, AND DR. V. PREDESCU

THE HISTORY OF RUMANIAN PSYCHIATRY

MEDICAL PSYCHIATRY IN RUMANIA began in the middle of the nine-teenth century. Prior to that time, and since antiquity, assistance to the mentally ill in the Rumanian principalities was given by the religious orders. The mentally ill were treated in certain monasteries designed for this purpose in Bucharest and Jassy, capitals of the principalities of Valachie and Maldavie, and in other places within these principalities, the union of which in 1859 was the origin of the present state of Rumania. The monks were charged with the mission of caring for the mentally ill, and they had special buildings constructed for this purpose.

In the ancient laws of Rumania can be found certain juridical norms that apply to the antisocial acts of the mentally ill, and among these laws appears the idea of medical intervention to identify the mentally ill. Thus, in the code of Volvade of Valachie, Mathieu Besarab (1652) under the title "The Signs of Insanity," one finds the following dispositions:

In order for the judge to recognize whether the person involved is truly insane, he interrogates the doctor who recognizes [the disorder] very easily.

The insane person, even if he commits a crime, will not be punished for it, but on the other hand will not be set free, lest he become a vagabond wandering throughout the country; he will be kept under constant surveillance until his reason returns to him.

Such prescriptions are proof of the advanced notions of this period: that the mentally ill were not criminally liable indicates that they were considered truly ill and in need of help, which was given them (notwithstanding their naïveté). Their confinement was superintended; reversal of psychic disorders was considered possible. The idea of medical care did not exist at this time. Especially in the seventeenth and eighteenth centuries the only steps taken toward treating those afflicted with mental illness were precautionary ones involving patients who were confined in monasteries for their offensive behavior. The patients, but above all their families, nourished the hope of a cure through divine intervention. This was particularly true in the monasteries, where there were icons reputed to have the power to effect spectacular "miracles."

Treatment was confined to reading and prayers and to a series of more or less solemn mystical ceremonies. These did not, however, end by condemning the patients to barbarous remedies, which was customary at that time in medieval Catholic Europe. This palpably more humane manner of treating the patients was noted by a number of travelers. The Catholic Archbishop, Marcus Bandinus, stresses the fact that the Jesuit priests who lived in the Rumanian principalities were astonished by the results obtained in hospitals for the "crazy" through gentle means and by prayer. (*Codex Bandinus, Annales Acad. Roum. Tome XVI, 1895.*)

Measures taken in western Europe for the care of the mentally ill at the beginning of the nineteenth century also had a salutary influence upon Rumania. Toward the end of 1838, the beginnings of formalized care for the mentally ill could be seen.

In the convent of Malamuci, near Bucharest, beggars had long been sheltered. In August, 1838, the ruling prince of the country, Alexander G. Ghica, decided that mental patients, as well as beggars, would be sent to Malamuci. Nine patients were then housed there. On December 11, 1838, the Minister of the Interior decided that assistance to the insane of Malamuci would become the responsibility of the "ephorie" (supervisor) of civilian hospitals.

It was then, for the first time, that medical assistance to mental patients actually became organized, through the nomination of a doctor and nurses capable of assuring scientific help, to the extent that the ideas and possibilities of the era allowed. From 1838 to 1845 the establishment of Malamuci, under the administration of the ephorie, functioned under these conditions.

In 1846 the treatment of patients, in the manner of the monasteries, passed into the charge of the "Department of the Faith." In this year the establishment of Malamuci was transferred to the monastery of Marcutza, where it was conducted from a medical point of view by Dr. Nicolas Ganasco. It housed 40 patients in 1847. In 1859 the number of patients increased to 100, and at the suggestion of Dr. Protici, Director of the hospital, a carpentry shop was created for the men and another shop of manual labor was developed for the women. Thus work therapy was first applied in Rumania at a rather early date.

In 1860 the Hospital for the Insane passed to the jurisdiction of the Ministry of the Interior, which became responsible for the organization of health in the country.

In April, 1864, the regulations of the Hospital of Marcutza were written and published in the *Medical Monitor* of the United Principalities, by the Inspector-General of the Health Service, Dr. Carol Davila. This document is important because it reflects the change from hygienic assistance of the monastic type to secular medical assistance. This change represents a qualitative step forward accomplished under the influence of the democratic bourgeois revolution which at this time was affirming its progressive, ascendant stage, struggling against the medieval organization then in a total decline.

The regulations reproduced the ideas of ancient Rumanian legislation, which maintained a policy of humanity and charity toward the patients (the "insane"), combined with the aspirations of the then current French philanthropy and that of the revolutionary Russian democrats. The author of this ruling, Dr. Carol Davila, who had been reared in France and had done his intellectual and medical studies there, warmly supported the democratic reforms achieved in Rumania by Prince Couze and his First Minister, Kogalniceanu. What had appeared in France in 1814 was the first interior regulation of a service for mental patients, which applied the ideas of Pinel and served as a model for all the services for the insane of France. From this ruling, Davila was able to deduce how the attributions of the medical service and the administrative service were established, and he adapted them to the specific exigencies of the United Principalities, putting them in accord with local customs.

The regulations of the hospital of Marcutza, which were hence to represent a conquest of reason and charity, comprised 114 articles grouped in seven chapters:

1. Functions of the Establishment
2. Entrance and Discharge of Patients
3. Interior Service of the Establishment
4. Dietary Regime
5. Bedding, Dress, and Measures of Cleanliness
6. Various Occupations and Rest
7. General Dispositions

The ruling of 1864 thus translated scientific rules of medical and administrative treatment into the practice of psychiatric care.

In 1866 the Hospital of Marcutza again passed to the administration of the Ephorie, now concerned solely with medical assistance to the sick, and thus the Ephorie was able to assure good organization for the mentally ill at this hospital. In 1867 the direction of the hospital of Marcutza was entrusted to Dr. Alexander Soutzo, who had made brilliant studies abroad and had a particular passion for psychiatry.

It was not until 1857 that The National School of Medicine and Pharmacy was created under the direction of Dr. Davila. In 1862, a course on mental illness was included in the curriculum.

In July, 1864, the University of Bucharest was founded by Royal decree and the School of Medicine became the Faculty of Medicine. This plan provided for a clinic of "mental illness" for the summer semester of the fifth (last) year. This clinic began in 1867–1868, on Sunday mornings at the Hospital of Marcutza, and was conducted by Dr. Soutzo. It was a free and voluntary course and was not incorporated into the faculty rules promulgated in 1871. The course continued in this form for ten years, until 1881, when Dr. Soutzo was named professor of legal medicine and toxicology. In 1893 the "mental clinic" became part of the official program of the faculty.

In 1897–1898, Professor Soutzo was appointed to the first Chair of Psychiatry and the Clinic of Mental Disorders. Dr. Mina Minovici was named assistant to the chair of legal medicine and in 1899 became its chief and inspiration.

Professor Alexander Soutzo (1837–1919) was virtually the founder of the school of Rumanian psychiatry. Endowed with energy and initiative, he dedicated himself to psychiatry with ardor. Through his publications and the medical reviews that he founded he laid the cornerstone of Rumanian medical literature. His publications *The Mentally Ill Confronting Life* and *Life and Matter* introduced the crucial materialist conception which characterized Rumanian Psychiatry during this period.

Professor Alexandre Obregia (1860–1937), who succeeded Soutzo to the chair of psychiatry at Bucharest, had worked for more than four years in the German clinics and the laboratories of Virchow, Munk, and Westphal, as well as in French hospitals with Charcot, Magnan, and Ball. In 1892, he was named Professor of Histology at the Faculty of Medicine at Bucharest, and in 1893 was named Chief Physician of the Hospital of Marcoutza. In 1910, Obregia was given the chair of the Clinic of Mental Illness. For twenty-four years (1910 to 1934), Professor Obregia was the leader of Rumanian psychiatry. Under his direction a descriptive specialty became a science in which the methods of clinical anatomy, experimentation, and biological analyses opened up unsuspected perspectives. Professor Obregia also realized the material conditions of the architectural and administrative order necessary for valuable scientific activity, as well as for superior medical assistance. As General Director of the Health Service, he created the Central Hospital of Mental Illness in Bucharest and the Hospital Socola de Jassy; he had the patients sent out of the monasteries, where they were isolated under some medical surveillance, and had them installed in the modern hospitals. The Central Hospital of Bucharest, inaugurated in 1923, was conceived as a vast establishment of pavilions in the middle of a park of several hectares at the edge of a village. Within its forty buildings, the mentally ill were treated under the best conditions of modern science. Today, this hospital is named after G. Marinesco, the founder of Rumanian neurology.

At the same time that Professor Obregia assumed direction of the chair of Bucharest, Professor Constantine I. Parhon was named to the Chair of Neurology and Psychiatry of Jassy, a great central university of Maldavia. A scientist of many capacities (biologist, neurologist, endocrinologist, and psychiatrist) resolutely taking a materialist and determinist stand, Professor Parhon created a veritable scientific center characterized by the same materialist orientation. He initiated study of the correlations between psychological troubles and endocrine disfunctions and of the problems of cerebral biochemistry. He focused on the material substratum of neuropsychic phenomena and considered that the bases of normal and pathological psychic life were to be found in functional and morphological biochemical modifications of the central nervous system, and he sought to study the way in which higher nervous activity determined them. Consideration of etiological factors resulting from the environment permitted Professor Parhon to consider the treatment of psychoses with optimism and thus to adopt a fundamentally different attitude from that of the majority of psychiatrists who thought that endogenous factors (hereditary) played a preponderantly fatal role in the genesis of mental illness. Professor Parhon thus continued and accentuated the traditional orientation of Rumanian psychiatry toward a positive therapeutic attitude. In 1909 he published, in collaboration with Goldstein, the first world-important publications on the glands of the internal secretions.

The organic and scientific development of Rumanian psychiatry is relatively recent. Before World War I, a series of works by Rumanian authors (Sutu, Obregia, Parhon, Urechia) described and interpreted various clinical cases, results of anatomical pathological research, results of various treatments, and results of research into secretions of the endocrine glands.

After World War I, the Society of Neurology and Psychiatry was founded. Until 1938 this society organized annual congresses in different parts of the country where psychiatric hospitals were located, and psychiatrists were given the opportunity to learn of each other's work and to debate the most important problems. In 1919, the Society edited a bulletin which published all the works of different centers of psychiatry and their findings and debates in the congress. This bulletin appeared until 1947.

During World War II, there was a relative stagnation in scientific psychiatric activity as well as in the activity of other medical fields. After the war, work was resumed in both organizational and scientific spheres. The communication sessions were reorganized in the cadre of the Society of Neurology and Psychiatry, but in the absence of a specialized journal they published only a few works of psychiatry in the *Review of Medical Sciences—Internal Medicine.*

A portion of the psychiatric studies in this period was collected in one volume called *Problems of Psychiatry* (1957) by the medical editor of Bucharest. These studies emphasize the weight of research regarding the material substratum of psychic troubles and the separation of the sub-specialties of child psychiatry, legal psychiatry, and organizational psychiatry from the preoccupation with the rehabilitation of psychic invalids. Psychiatric activity was developed still further with the appearance in 1956 of an organ of publicity for the specialty and with the reorganization of the conferences and annual reunions, the first of which took place at Bucharest in 1955.

Since the war a great number of studies have focused on neuroses, especially on neuroasthenia appearing after certain nervous activity. In addition to clinical description and considerations of the role of environmental factors, there have been numerous studies of psychosomatic modifications such as those caused by the endocrines. Clinical and laboratory observations led to the conclusion of the existence of states of hyperthyroidism, hyperfolliculinemia, hypoparathyroidism, and adrenal hypofunction. The presence of seventeen ketosteroids in the urine of the neurasthenic consistently showed an appreciable deviation from the normal, either of more or of less, which made definitive conclusions impossible.

Potassium, calcium, cholesterol, and glutathion determinations have also been carried out, and it has been found that a number of different mental states were included in the diagnosis of neurasthenia; the limits of this diagnosis thus tended to become extended to an unwarranted degree. The errors of diagnosis were found to consist in the confusion of the neurasthenia due to (nervous) overtaxation with endocrine disorders, involutional disturbances, and with asthenia appearing after craniocerebral traumatism or after somatic, toxic, or infectious disorders. This discovery has led to the search for specific criteria to delimit nervous asthenia. In this direction, some work has appeared on the erroneous interpretation of the notion of neuroses and on the delimitation of the category of neurasthenia, which must be considered as such only when it is due to psychogenic factors and when no symptoms of organicity appear in the foreground. This holds even if the appearance of symptoms is primarily due to psychogenic factors (as for example Basedow's postemotional disorder). Nevertheless, we have not discounted predisposing factors such as those of the endocrine, certain somatic ailments which constitute the argument that favors the asthenia of (nervous) overtaxation.

As elsewhere, schizophrenia is a major concern. One investigator, C. Csiky, hypothesized the existence of a process affecting certain morphofunctional structures which had been weakened by predisposing, favoring and provoking factors. P. Brinzei regards schizophrenia as an encephelodystrophy of a endoexogenous nature. Others distinguish true schizophrenia from schizophrenic syndromes of pseudoschizophrenias. There is a tendency to accept a polyetiology of diagnostic states in general as "schizophrenia" and to differentiate true schizophrenia from the schizophrenic-type disorders. There have also been numerous biochemical and electroencephalographic investigations. Studies on ephatic functions, by the method of Leeper and Vespi (provoked hyperglycemia), lead to the conclusion of a lowering of the tolerance of glucose—a fact observed also by several foreign writers. They note however, that modifications in glucose metabolism can also be due to other factors. Investigating the blood of schizophrenics led to the notion of an oxidation deficiency. Brinzei and his collaborators studied the distribution of I^{131} and p^{32} in the organism and the fluids of schizophrenics. Meiu and his collaborators determined the cereuloplasmin, copper, and glutothione in the afferent and efferent blood in the brain and in the venous blood of general circulation (the method of Myerson and Hachbran); they established in the venous blood of the brain, in relation to the peripheral blood, an enlarged content of ceruloplasmin, copper, and total reduced glutothione and a lessening of oxidized glutothione.

Csiky and Sciky-Wagner conducted hemotological research and, finding the eosinemia increased, they interpreted it as an immunobiological weakness of the organism; this finding appears in recent processes and in the phases of recrudescence, decreasing in a manner parallel to clinical remission. That the augmentation of the eosinemia disappears in the chronic forms shows a part of the aggressiveness of external noxious factors; the presence of these is proven, according to the authors, by a retardation in the maturation of visible elements as ascertained on the basis of slides taken from the sternum.

Electroencephalographic and pneumoencephalographic studies were made by V. Predescu and his collaborators, who found normal traces in 33.65 percent of the cases they studied and pathological traces in 66.35 percent. The highest number of normal traces occur in the stage of repeated remission, whereas the lowest number occur in chronic defective schizophrenics. In one group of patients they found a reaction toward the different stimulants. Among certain cases these investigators also carried out pneumoencephalograms; the radiological changes were either of the atrophy type or of the ventricular modiciation type. In correlating the electroencephalographic data with such pneumoencephalographic data they found bioeletric alterations in 72 percent of the cases of pathological pneumoencephalograms. Arginteru and Aurelia Sirbu found that the most important electroencephalographic alterations were encountered during the progressive phases, and they decreased correspondingly with the phenomena of compensation. The authors did not remark parallelism between electric modifications and clinical ones.

In casting a general glance on the results of the researches concerning the physiopathology of schizophrenia, we note that although these were not always superimposed on one another, certain ones among them appeared with greater frequency. These are: (1) the presence of certain toxic substances; (2) the frequent functional lowering of certain organs, endocrine glands, metabolism; (3) the lowering of the reactivity and of the possibility of adaptation; (4) the return to normal of certain indices, pathologically modified, parallel with clinical amelioration—facts which demonstrate that the respective disorders are truly part of the background of pathological processes.

THE PSYCHIATRY OF OLD AGE

The Psychiatry of Old Age is also an object of some research. C. I. Parhon and his colleagues found, in a decreasing order of frequency, stereotypes in language and movement, thought disturbances, instability and impulsiveness, a reactive depression, bulimia, memory trouble and trouble with attention.

Among the conclusions of this work we note again the increased frequency of arteriosclerosis among old people with psychic troubles, the favorable influence of thyroid treatment, of treatment with novocain and vitamin E, of work and of family life; and on the other hand, we found the unfavorable influence of life in a group composed exclusively of old people, and of retirement, which needs to be adapted to the psychic and physical capacity of the aged.

Constanta Parhon-Stefanescu, Elena Preda, and Felicia Cherciulescu carried out biochemical research determining glutathion, iron, copper, hemoglobin, and the number of corpuscles in the blood of senile psychotics, as compared with the blood of psychologically normal men of the same age; disturbances in the normal proportions of these constant elements lead to the conclusion that the process of oxidation is insufficient and that the resistance of the organisms lowered, as in the appearance of certain mechanisms of compensation (the augmentation of corpuscles, of iron, and of copper). The same authors find among senile psychotics, as compared with normal men of the same age, an augmentation of the ratio of proteins to lipids to the detriment of the decreasing lipids. This is perhaps due to certain deposits of lipids in the tissues as well as to a lower solubility of these among the senile psychotics. In a work concerning the general aspects of the psychiatry of the aged, Constanta Parhon-Stefanescu concludes that in senile dementia the pathological and morphofunctional phenomena which appear after a certain age are exacerbated. Given the diversity of involutional psychoses, the author believes that a division of involutional psychoses into "dementing" and "nondementing" is more realistic than the classical division into the forms of presenile and senile dementia.

In the areas of psychoses due to vascular disturbances, we note the work of V. Predescu, who tried to establish certain criteria of diagnosis that distinguish between chronic arteriosclerotic psychoses and senile psychoses with hallucinatory-delirious phenomena. The first appear later and do not present any distinguishing phenomena of dementia; the auditory hallucinations are vivid, persisting, and connected primarily with the development of delirious ideas. We note also the work of A. Retezennu, and his colleagues, who showed certain common symptoms in the clinical picture, i.e., psychomotor agitation and anxiety underlying a confusional syndrome; ideas of prejudice, depression, and hallucinations appear simultaneously with clinical improvement. The authors explained the appearance of psychic disturbances as a metabolic error connected with the anoxia of the cortical and subcortical nerve cells.

Continuing the tradition of the school of Professor Parhon, many researchers have tried to present evidence of the connection between psychic and endocrine disturbances. In this area we note the publication of cases regarding certain manic-depressive patients in whom the attacks disappeared following thyroidectomy; at that time it was shown that this therapeutic method did not always give good results, and in certain it was ineffective, which shows that the pathogenic mechanism of the manic-depressive psychosis is not always the same.

Several cases of mental disturbances were published, such as anxiety, the catatonic states, and the maniacal syndromes appearing on top of hyperthyroidism. In order to extend their knowledge of the pathogenesis of psychic disturbances of hyperthyroidism, Constanta Parhon-Stefanescu, Elena Prada, and Florica Meiu undertook research on the chemistry of the afferent and efferent blood of the brain among hyperthyroid dogs. Compared with the control animals, the brains of animals treated with the thyroid extract retained less, or even lost, component glucose, retained potassium, and lost magnesium and phosphorous.

A series of psychopathological problems were then treated: euphoria, the post-schizophrenic personality, perception in the esthenic and depressive state, and thought disturbances among stabilized schizophrenics.

The majority of recent works on therapy concern experience with neuroplegics, but even more remarkable methods have been found for treatment of epilepsy by using eserine and the treatment of serious acute mental states by use of blood transfusion. Some works have been devoted to the capacity of the mentally ill to work, to their preparation in the occupational therapy situation, and to the possibilities of rehabilitation.

Child psychiatry in Rumania, neglected as a special branch of psychiatry until the end of World War II, began to be developed in the last decade and was made a formal branch by the organization (mentioned above) of the first conference of Neurology, Psychiatry, and Endocrinology. Many works have appeared concerning psychiatric care of the mentally ill child, clinical aspects, therapy, etc. Among these we note the care of children with psychic and neurological troubles; studies on the prevention of children's mental disorders, in which emphasis is placed on the importance of hours of conversation with the parents and field work outside the consultation service (foyers, schools, nurseries); adequate therapeutic measures for different age groups; possible applications of prophylaxis of psychic disorders among children by examining the parents, protecting the mother during pregnancy, the possibility of following the child's development, assuring the child good living conditions, correcting endocrine troubles, treating every abnormal psychic symptom. The prevention of extreme aftereffects of the child's cerebral lesions is being studied in a sample group of 200 children between one and sixteen years. The authors specially emphasize post-traumatic effects, showing that it is important to exclude as evidence children who have suffered traumas.

Additional work in the field of child psychiatry include articles on neuroses, general paralysis, and schizophrenia among children.

LEGAL PSYCHIATRY

As we have shown above, the beginnings of legal psychiatry in our country appeared long ago, and elements of this field are to be found in the archives of the seventeenth-century law.

The current legislation of Rumania recognizes the necessity of psychiatric expertise in cases where some doubt exists as to the sanity of a lawbreaker or a person who has broken a contract. In the case of uncertainty, a supplementary testimony of experts is admitted; moreover, each party has the right to designate a counselor who shares the expertise.

As to penal problems, Article 128 of The Rumanian Penal Code states that a person is ". . . not answerable for an act committed during a state of unconsciousness caused by mental derangement or other causes."

If the violator is considered mentally ill to such a degree that he is incapable of understanding the exigencies of the law, that he is unaware of the cause of his actions, that he cannot evaluate the seriousness of his acts or foresee their consequences, or that he is incapable of controlling his conduct, he is absolved from legal punishment, and only therapeutic measures are recommended for him. In a case where such a violator is dangerous to society, the penal code provides for "measures of security." These (measures) are indicated in Articles 71, 72, and 73. They consist of confining the sick in a special institution designed for this purpose, in a special section of a hospital for the mentally ill, or in an institution of rehabilitation. Confinement in these institutions ends when the patient is no longer considered dangerous. If the patient is harmless, he is either kept in an ordinary section of a hospital for the mentally ill, or is left to the care and custody of his family.

In our country there is such a hospital for special observation where, beside treatment, closer attention is given. One can consider, always as a measure of security, the steps taken recently to provide for the obligatory confinement of patients who present a serious social danger, meaning those who are dangerous to themeslves or who endanger the life or health of others, or those who may commit serious infractions of the law. The treatment may allow the patient to be ambulatory or may require his confinement. The institution or cessation of treatment is decided by judicial request with the advice of medical councils as indicated in decree number 12 of January 27, 1965.

Article 65 of the Code of Penal Procedure provides for the possibility of suspending judgment or punishment in the case of mental derangement, that is, when during the trial the violator is found to be in a condition described by Article 128 of the Penal Code.

If infractions have been committed in the state of inebriety caused by alcohol, by other toxic substances, or by drugs, mentioned in article 129 of the Penal Code, the person is not considered responsible when his inebriation is due to "certain circumstances entirely unforeseen by the author of the infraction and completely independent of his volition." The law provides for a one-fifth reduction in the penalty for the violator if he committed the infraction during "a state of complete drunkenness"; this reduction is not granted if it is proved that the violator intentionally brought on his state of inebriety with the aim either of lessening his punishment or of facilitating his commission of the crime. In this case the infraction is considered to be premeditated. It is worth noting that nowhere in the law is pathological intoxication mentioned; in practice, however, profound disturbances of conscience are taken into account and Article 128 applies to the violator. Article 129 is not applied in cases of traffic accidents caused by intoxication. These are discussed in a special article of the Penal Code. Acts of sexual perversion and acts of "bestiality" ("perversion between man and animals") are similarly punishable by law.

The counsel of the Commissions of Judicial Psychiatry, ordinarily composed of two medical psychiatrists and a medical lawyer, is often sought in order to establish civil incapacity and cause for indictment (Article 142 of the Family Code) or with a view toward lifting an indictment in a situation where the causes that provoked it have ceased to operate.

Insofar as the mental patient is deemed incapable of carrying out contracts, his marriage is prohibited by the law (Article 9 of the Family Code). The request for separation (divorce) from a mental patient is granted by our laws, which even specify that the separation implies no attempt at reconciliation, if it is based on (the patient's) chronic mental illness.

Patients with mental disorders, as well as minors below the age of 15, cannot act as witnesses when evidence is presented in trials of infractions (Articles 136 of the Code of Penal Procedure), but they may be interrogated as informants without being under oath (Article 145 of the Code of Penal Procedure).

Confinement of mental patients, except those who present a serious social threat, is carred out in the same manner as for those with somatic disorders, as has been shown above.

The legislation with regard to minors provides for the irresponsibility of minors up to 12 years, responsibility up to 15 years only if it is felt that the minor committed the punishable deed with full awareness of what he was doing and, after 15 years, the minor is considered responsible to the same extent as the adult (Article 139 of the Penal Code). The law emphasizes the necessity for legal proceedings to take into account information concerning the minor's physical state, his guardians, the conditions under which he has grown up and lived, and the moral and material situation of his family. Depending on his mental state, the minor is sent either to a hospital or to an institute for rehabilitation.

As in other countries, the existence or nonexistence of diminished responsibility and the ability or inability of the doctor to pronounce on the responsibility or irresponsibility of people with mental disorders are continuing issues. The legislation in Rumania does not provide for diminished responsibility, but does provide for extenuating circumstances, such as cases in which "the infraction was committed under the influence of a strong emotion." Psychiatrists are divided in their opinions as to what constitutes the criteria for recognizing diminished responsibility. Thus E. Pamfil supports the existence of diminished responsibility, because ". . . man cannot be divided into two perfectly distinct categories on the one hand, normal and responsible people, and on the other, completely irresponsible, disturbed individuals; between these two types is one represented by the unstable." E. Tomerug believes it necessary to admit many degrees, such as complete responsibility, diminished responsibility and irresponsibility. P. Brinzei has noted that difficulty arises from the fact that certain medical experts go beyond the scientific limits of psychiatry in proceeding to a formal declaration on "penal" responsibility, although certain situations necessitate a reduction in penal responsibility.

Whether a doctor should pronounce on the responsibility of the [mentally] ill was discussed in 1962 at the Conference of Judicial Psychiatry held in Bucharest. The majority of the committee was of the opinion that psychiatric experts should not decide responsibility but should only describe psychic symptomatology, on the basis of which the diagnosis and the relationship between mental suffering and danger from a social point of view are established. Then on the basis of these decisions is built the ability to discern the person who has undergone the expert examination.

In the area of the scientific activity of legal psychiatry, we note the earlier work of Parhon and then that of Minovici and Stanescu in which the determinism of crime and the constitution of the criminal are considered, and the work of Kernbach, who was concerned with the problem of [legal] responsibility, etc.

Among the more recent works, in addition to those already mentioned, are those that discuss the following problems: responsibility of the mentally ill in general, the expert valuation of judicial psychiatry or various types of illness. Thus we note the work of Brinzei and his collaborators in which they show the frequency of dangerous implications, from a social point of view, of schizophrenia—in relation to the form of the illness—and the difficulties encountered in establishing a retrospective critical judgment among the schizoid psychopaths, among whom psychotic elements temporarily appear under conditions of certain psychic traumas. E. Tomerug and his collaborators are interested in the medico-legal aspects of schizophrenia in relation to the clinical form of the illness. Expert judgment becomes difficult in cases that involve beginning schizophrenia, a form of this illness in which the symptoms can pass unrecognized ("latent schizo-phrenia"). Parhon-Stefanescu and E. Tomerug have sought to establish criteria of responsibility for those suffering from craniotrauma, because they often have behavioral disorders which may be compensated for under hospital conditions. The authors conclude that they can establish with probability a connection between trauma and the psychic trouble which has led to the infraction of the law when the trauma has occurred in a young individual, neurological signs of epilepsy appear, there is a great loss of bone and cerebral substance, and there is not too great an interval between the trauma and the moment when the infraction was committed. The authors also concern themselves with the infractions and the respon-sibility of those with cerebral arteriosclerosis.

Finally, a few works have been devoted to violations of the law by minors. Thus E. Tomerug and his collaborators proposed that a record for juvenile violators be set up in a center for observation of minors, in which they will be studied in every aspect by a committee of experts composed of a child psychiatrist, a psychologist, and an endocrinologist. Only with such dossier should a minor be sent up for legal proceedings. The authors emphasize the importance of the action in directing these minors toward a center of education or of medical surveillance.

In the same area P. Brinzei and his collaborators propose an expert study of every juvenile violator by a medical-judiciary psychiatric com-mittee in collaboration with a psychopedagogue.

For the prevention of juvenile delinquency, the authors propose, among other measures, setting up records on every child with mental or moral defects manifested in the course of the school period and afterwards, up to majority, in the background of the social life of the young.

THE TEACHING OF PSYCHIATRY

Psychiatry occupies an important place in the complex of general medical knowledge, if we keep in mind that this specialty, studied together with the other branches of medicine, gives medical students the oppor-tunity to better comprehend the concept of illness as representing an inter-ruption in the organism's adaptation to the conditions of its environment. In the light of this conception, defense and adaptation reactions are under-stood through their dynamic nature, in a unified way, and offer students the premises for forming an evolutionist understanding and at the same time a conviction of the general aspect of morbid states. This conviction will always serve to make the future doctor aware of the concept that the organism is an internally unified whole which is found in turn in its complex dynamic unity with the environment. In this way we accord to psychiatry (which in Rumania is taught in the sixth year) the prestigious task of curbing the tendency to compartmentalize human pathology. These tendencies are due to the material situation of modern medicine, which is characterized by the trend toward very narrow specialization, even within a single specialty. Under the conditions of the general [extern or non-resident, hospital] studentship (put into practice in 1964) medical students have an opportunity to solidly assimilate the principal disciplines of practice in sections (medical, surgical, obstetrical and gynecological, infectious-contagious diseases, etc.). Thus, before proceeding to the study of psychiatry, students already have had the opportunity to develop their thoughts concerning other specialties in regard to function and prophylaxis.

The teaching of psychiatry is organized in such a way that it offers students the opportunity to be convinced once more that in the great majority of cases of human pathology dynamic-functional troubles play a preponderant role. Most particularly, psychiatric instruction has the mission of convincing them that the narrowly localized anatomist conception, as much in psychiatry as in other specialties, does not correspond to reality and that only the dynamic functional conception can explain the complexity of interactions and reciprocal conditions of mechanisms of psychic or neurovegetative-endocrine activity. The study of psychiatry helps students surmount the mechanistic [notion of] monocausality and obliges them to return with conviction to the dialectic unity of the interaction of exterior and interior factors; moreover, this study requires students to analyze not only the clinical picture and the etiology, but also the special conditions under which the latter operates. These conditions include the particular reactions of the nervous system, the somatic state of the individual and particularly the aspects of the determinist, unitary, individual-environmental context in general and the social environment in particular. By following a similar line of reasoning, we give very particular attention to the study of hereditary and constitutional factors, the latter being regarded as a dynamic complex of innate and acquired factors. As for the formation of character and personality, the preponderant role is accorded to the social environment.

In this connection we emphasize that in the function of the environment in general, and the social environment in particular, several biological deficiencies, or hereditary acquired deficiencies, can appear exacerbated or reduced.

As is made clear in the account of the historical psychiatric problems in Rumania and in the enumeration of the areas of Rumanian scientific research, the important interests of these psychiatrists are directed toward the study of the material substratum which is the basis of mental disorders. The principal tendency in the orientation of Rumanian psychiatry consists in enriching the possibilities of a solid foundation of psychiatric nosology to establish criteria capable of differentiating mental disorders and, as a function of this, preventative measures, early detection, and adequate treatment. At the same time, the selection and application of different methods used in the complex effort of reintroducing the mentally ill into society constitutes one of the constant and considerable preoccupations of Rumanian psychiatry.

In Rumania the teaching of psychiatry takes on the following forms according to the aim and audience to which it is addressed:

1. Teaching psychiatry with a view toward the complex education of students at the Faculty of General Medicine, Pediatrics, and Stomatology.

2. Teaching psychiatry designed for the faculty of Specialization and Advanced Training.

3. Teaching psychiatry as it is taught to students is practiced on the level of psychiatric clinics belonging to the university centers of Bucharest, Jassy, Clui, Timisoara, and Tirgu-Mures. These clinics are directed to the didactic and scientific point of view by the collective disciplines or (collective) chairs of psychiatry.

4. Postgraduate instruction in psychiatry is provided at the Faculty of Specialization and at the Faculty of Advanced Study of the Institute of Medicine and Pharmacy. Admission to the course of specialization at these faculties is achieved following a competitive examination for psychiatric intern posts in hospitals after a period of general medical practice or a minimum of three years' residency in psychiatry.

Psychiatry is taught differently (in the sixth year) to students of the Faculty of Pediatrics and to those of the Faculty of General Medicine. First, this differentiation is by the contents of the plan of instruction, i.e., at the Faculty of Pediatrics primary emphasis is placed on the child's psychomotor development and next on particular aspects of the psychology and psychopathology of the child, and finally on his mental disorders. Second, in order that theoretical instruction be more closely linked to the medical practice of future pediatricians, a six-week nonresident (extern) hospital term was introduced in 1964 in the Faculty of Pediatrics. During this term, sixth-year students are obliged to work four hours a day in the child psychiatry sections of the psychiatric clinic, to learn the aspects of neuropsychiatric pathology in greater depth and to treat them. The extern students each have to take care of a minimum of between five and ten patients. The diagnosis and treatment of these patients are established by the body of instructors in charge of directing the students. During this period the teaching staff responsible for the activity of the extern students organize discussions on the diagnosis of each case, arrange presentations of clinical cases on the collective level of the chair for the more complex cases, and oversee sessions during which reports are presented by the students that deal with subjects chosen by the instructing groups. Initially, the extern term at the Faculty of Pediatrics was intended to provide all future pediatricians with the opportunity to gain a more solid knowledge of pathological aspects of child development, to know how to recognize and combat the easier and more common pathologies, and to manage in a qualified manner those cases that go beyond the profile and the possibilities of ambulatory or hospital treatment. Thus this program consolidates, in fact, the basis of a precocious prophylactic orientation in order to anticipate the psychic troubles of adolescents or of the adults of tomorrow. There remains, however, the desideratum of extending the extern student term in the future to the Faculty of General Medicine, where, because of the very heavy teaching load, it has not been possible to provide an extern term for students. At the Faculty of General Medicine the students pursue clinical instruction in psychiatry and practical demonstrations during the first semester of the sixth year. But for the interns of the Faculty of General Medicine who want to specialize in psychiatry, there is the opportunity of undergoing a six-month internship at the psychiatric clinic.

The program of instruction in psychiatry for the Faculty of Stomatology is more limited and is directed toward completing the medical culture of students in stomatology; they study psychiatry in their fourth year.

Interns who have been in practice for at least two years after completing their study at the Institute of Medicine and Pharmacy are also admitted to this course. Here interns are defined as those doctors who, during their internship training, have completed at least a six-month term in psychiatric and neurological clinics. Until they achieve the title of medical specialist in psychiatry, those doctors who succeed in the psychiatric interns competition in the hospitals specialize in this field for a minimum of three years.

Psychiatric internship in the hospitals is worked out in the following way: During the first year all psychiatric interns take certain clinical courses and practice in the university clinics. The majority of interns complete their three-year internship in the clinical hospitals at the university centers of Bucharest, Jassy, Clouj, Timichoire, and Tirgou-Moureche. At the end of these three years the psychiatric interns are allowed to present themselves for examinations for certification. Designation of the title of psychiatrist and a position in a particular part of the country is decided on the basis of a competition. The winners are awarded the vacant posts, which are announced in advance by the press prior to the competition.

However, acquisition of knowledge does not end with the examinations and the competition for the title or position of medical specialist in psychiatry. Thus a three- to four-month proficiency course has been organized by the Faculty of Specialization and Advanced Study. This course allows medical specialists to enrich and revive their theoretical and practical knowledge, and offers them the opportunity of being in direct contact with the methods and scientific concerns of the university clinics.

After eight years of practice in psychiatry and a minimum of ten years in the field of health, medical specialists in psychiatry are eligible for certification and competition for the title of chief (primary) doctor, and vacant posts, announced in the press, are awarded.

Special proficiency courses for chief doctors are also offered at the level of the faculties spoken of above. These courses last from two to four months.

To promote the assimilation of fundamental notions, the program of instruction for doctors and pharmacists at the Faculty of Specialization and Advanced Study gives certain three- to four-month courses for neurologists who work in the general polyclinics where they often encounter a good number of nervous disorders, disharmonies, and even psychic difficulties. Two- to three-month courses of initiation also have been given for psychologists and *logopèdes* who work in the departments of psychiatry and child psychiatry of the general polyclinics. It should be mentioned that specialization and perfection of skills in the fields of adult and child psychiatry are achieved in a distinct and different way.

ASSISTANCE AND ORGANIZATION

Hospital care is assured with the help of 12,000 beds for psychiatric patients, and the network of psychiatry hospitals is developing all the time. This improved situation can be readily appreciated if one knows that in 1938 in Rumania there were not more than 4,211 beds for psychiatric patients, whereas, presently more than 12,000 beds are available. Rumania's system of child neuropsychiatry was founded and developed rapidly along with the system of ambulatory care in departments of active consultation. This system includes more than 150 specialized departments.

Care of the acutely ill, whom the state requires to be hospitalized, is provided in psychiatric hospitals and in the psychiatric wards of general hospitals. For neurotic patients, special wards are provided in psychiatric hospitals and sanitariums.

For patients who exhibit prolonged psychic effects, or for chronic patients, there are hospitals and special wards where particular emphasis is placed on pharmacological therapy and especially on the intense activity of socially rehabilitating patients. This is done with the help of work therapy methods applied in diverse workshops, with the intermediary of agricultural trades.

Psychiatric care of children is carried out separately. Sometimes there are small psychiatric wards in a separate circuit that are organized in the heart of pediatric hospitals. Children who exhibit neuropsychic conditions are hospitalized in special institutions, which are called "nursery-hospitals." Children in these institutions benefit as much from specialized (psychiatric) care as from pedagogic instruction and work therapy, depending on their degree of accessibility, retardation, or psychic defectiveness.

For children who show mental deficiency, whatever the degree, or a mild form of imbecility, there are special boarding schools where, according to the degree of retardation, the principal emphasis is placed on education or on assimilation of work habits.

In these schools such children pursue the possibility of qualifying for various trades, depending on the potential and aptitude of each child. Admission to nursery-asylums and special schools is approved by complex committees which include child psychiatric and psychological specialists. Depending on the case (if it is a matter of sensory, motor, or endocrine deficiencies), an appeal is made to other groups (O.R.I.-ists, orthopedists or endocrinologists, etc.). Ambulatory care of children is provided by teams of specialists (child psychiatrists, psychologists, logopèdes, social workers, or sisters in pediatrics). It should be mentioned that active consultation is offered in all these departments.

The medical hygiene staff of the departments of child psychiatry is closely linked to the collectives for preschool children (nurseries, day nurseries, nursery schools, children's homes, public schools, etc.). Doctors of the communities, school doctors, and public health specialists jointly study the conditions in which these communities operate and bring out the environmental aspects which encourage illness.

In Rumania the administration and variety of hospitals have in common their state auspices and the gratuitousness of the assistance granted to the ill. The system according to which hospitals and psychiatric wards are built is that of pavilions. More than 80 percent of hospitalized patients do not receive care in closed rooms. The care for those patients who are acutely disturbed, in danger of trying to escape, or of committing aggressive acts toward themselves or others is provided in closed rooms where they are assured constant surveillance during the entire acute phase, after which the patients are transferred to rooms with open doors in the same pavilion.

The circuit necessary for psychiatric patients is afforded by a complex functional liaison between pavilions. Thus, certain patients who have committed serious antisocial acts are transferred to a pavilion specially designed for the problems of psychiatric-judicial expertise. Cases of general progressive paralysis or where there is suspicion of neurosyphilis accompanying psychic disturbances are transferred to a pavilion where, in addition to regular treatments, specific treatments are applied (e.g., fever therapy and, in particular, malaria therapy). Patients can also change their pavilion of treatment if they manifest a desire to be treated by another doctor. Transfer of patients for a special sleep cure is provided for a period of 16 to 20 days, after which they return to their initial pavilions. There is a positive and absolutely necessary functional liaison between work-therapy pavilions and other pavilions of the hospital. In case of decompensation or relapse of patients in work-therapy pavilions, transfer is made to other psychiatric pavilions, and, inversely, patients in psychiatric pavilions are transferred to work-therapy pavilions when they have improved sufficiently for gradual work.

In general, it is considered necessary to transfer to work therapy those mental patients whose state of improvement is not sufficient for them to return to their families. In these cases, work therapy, in combination with uninterrupted pharmacological treatment and a convalescent regimen characteristic of these pavilions, gradually brings about the possibility of social rehabilitation and permits the patient to leave the hospital. But in certain cases where therapeutic results become evident in a shorter period of time, and patients may not stay in the hospital except to undergo work therapy, they live confined in the same pavilion, undergo treatment every day, go to workshops for work therapy and afterward return to the pavilion. In our hospitals, as elsewhere, discussions are organized among treating doctors, work-therapy doctors, and instructors of work therapy in order to keep in touch with the patient's behavior during work and to appreciate as a group the quality of his development, as well as the outlook for his social rehabilitation.

In general, the activity of psychiatric hospitals is coordinated by a director and—depending on the number of beds—by one or two associate directors, an administrator, and a group administrator. In dealing with technical problems, the hospital director collaborates fully with the (administrative) hospital council, which includes the heads of wards, of pavilions, and—for psychiatric hospital clinics—of didactic groups as well. This council convenes at the director's indication whenever necessary. On these occasions an analysis is made of the quality of the treatment being offered, the problems of scientific research are established, and measures designed to improve the functioning of the hospital are debated.

Hospital care is provided by medical teams and auxiliary personnel of average qualifications. Each pavilion is directed by a doctor-in-chief (primary) psychiatrist who has seniority in his work and experience, and clinical pavilions are directed by a didactic staff. Other primary doctors or psychiatric specialists and interns at the psychiatric hospitals are also part of the staff of the doctor-in-chief of the pavilion, so that there is a doctor for every twenty to twenty-five beds. In the clinical pavilions, given the increased number of didactic tasks, there is a doctor for every twelve to fifteen beds. In the staff of a pavilion there are also medical assistants (who have finished high school and then a three-year school for medical qualification), [Catholic] medical sisters, nurses and nurses' aides. The job scheme of psychiatric hospitals also provides for groups of psychologists, mechanotherapists, and social workers who contribute greatly to this activity of health care. These groups are guided by the hospital administration, which in turn is aided by the heads of wards and pavilions.

In Rumania special emphasis is placed, from the beginning of hospitalization, on conditions necessary for better social readaptation of patients after their release from the hospital. With a view toward achieving these desiderata, groups of social workers directed by the heads of the pavilion seek to discover certain basic facts about the patients: the family, the place of residence, the place of work and, if necessary, certain legal complications. Thus, release from the hospital takes place only when the patient's state of mental health permits it and when the patient's social problems have been wholly or at least greatly resolved. When patients belong to a department where there is an out-patient system (active consultation), the patient's dossier is sent to the department of active consultation at the time he is discharged from the hospital. The dossier contains a great deal of information, diagnosis, clinical facts, state of health at the time the patient left the hospital, indications of ambulatory treatment, medical leave taken from work, resumption of work and other social problems that is designed to assure cured patients easier social readaptation. When the departments of active consultation are too distant for the patient to reach, handling of interviews [therapy] is carried out under the observation of doctors of the health district, and periodic specialized inspection is again the duty of the doctors administering treatment or of consultation services outside the departmental or regional psychiatric hospital.

In chronic cases, hospitals for acute patients are responsible for directing them to chronic wards and are obliged at the same time to send the ticket of transfer and the records of pharmacological therapy, work therapy, and symptoms denoting the illness as observed during the patient's stay at the hospital.

Patients having high potential for infractions and those who have already committed serious acts are handled in the same way as the chronic cases, and are sent to hospitals specially designed for this type of patient. But then the transfer cannot be carried out except following a judicial order which is based on the conclusions of the psychiatric-judicial expert report.

In order to coordinate and scientifically support the activity of psychiatric medical care, the Minister of Health and Social Prevention (M.S.P.S.) created a psychiatric methodological council, including highly qualified psychiatrists, psychologists, and social workers. On the initiative and advice of the M.S.P.S. and with a view toward elaborating the materials necessary to develop and improve the care given to psychiatric cases, this council moves about the country and organizes conferences which deal with problems of health care at the regional level and the city level, and discuss departmental centers.

During the popular-democratic regime favorable conditions were created for solving questions of care to the mentally ill. In addition to the rapid increase in the number of beds for psychiatric patients, the network of specialized territorial polyclinics has grown each year. This network provides qualified, accessible, and free ambulatory care. To detect mental disturbances at early stages the polyclinics collaborate with the health personnel of the health districts, school and business doctors, and teachers at all school levels. Economic measures, instructive educational measures, and the general organization of medical care effectively contribute to the development of the mental health of the population and to the prevention of mental illness. The method of active consultation (therapy) has been extended, to provide for early detection of symptoms, to assure appropriate ambulatory treatment, to direct patients in time to appropriate institutions, to put them under surveillance and to continually guide cases discharged from the hospital, to create favorable conditions of work and of life in the social environment, and to put preventative measures into practice on a large scale. Such well-organized active consultation will in time limit the need for hospitalization, thus freeing hospital beds.

The chair of psychiatry at the Institute of Medico-Pharmacy operates in the hospital headed by Professor Dr. Gh. Marinesco and is currently directed by Professor Dr. Constanta Parhon-Stefanescu.

References

1. D. ARGINTERU AND AURELIA SIRBU: "Problems corelatiilor electroclinice in schizofrenie." Conf. Nationala de Psihiatrie, Bucuresti, 1964.
2. I. BALLIF, S. BLUMENFELD, AND G. MEIU: "Problems de organizer a neuropsihiatriei infantile." Prima Conefatuire pe tara de neurologie, psihiatrie si endocrinologie infantila (Remumatele repoartelor), Iasi, 1958.
3. C. BELCIUGATEANU: "Euforia din cursul nevrozelor." *Neurologie, Psihiatrie, Neurochirurgia*, 2, 115, 1962.
4. C. BELCIUGATEANU: "Cerecterul in cadrul psihopstiilor." *Neur., Psih., Neurochir.*, 5, 453, 1963.
5. C. BELCIUGATEANU AND S. DIACICOV: "Depresiunes in cadrul nevrozeier." *Neur., Psih., Neurochir.*, 3, 223, 1964.
6. S. BLUMENFELD, I. STRACHINARU, AND C. ROMANESCU: "Cu privire la problems profilexiei balilor psihiceale copilului." *Neur., Psih., Neurochir.*, 5, 389, 1957.
7. S. BLUMENFELD AND ANGELA SUTU: "Problema prevenirii tulburarilor psihice ale copilului si cadrul posibilitatilor ei practice de realizare." Prima Consfatuire pe tara de neurologie, psihiatrie si endocrinologie infantila, Iasi, 1958.
8. S. BLUMENFELD, B. PALINGER, J. AVREMOVICI, AND E. L. PENDEFUNDA: Studiul clinic si experimental in paralizie generala infantila. "Probleme de Psihiatrie," Ed. Medicolo, Bucuresti, 1951.
9. P. BRINZEI, C. ROMANESCU, I. STREICHMAN, AND C. BARBU: "Consideratii asupre rolului defectivitatii psihice infantile juvenile in generaree actelor socialmento periculcese." *Neur., Psih., Neurochir.*, 3, 267, 1963.
10. P. BRINZEI: "Consideretii asupre responsabilitatii penale atenuate a bolnavil or psihici." *Neur., Psih., Neurochir.*, 4, 1963.
11. P. BRINZEI, N. PARUS, T. PIROZYASKI, P. BERBA, AND GH. SCRIPEARU: Consideretiuni asupra implicatiilor judiciare a bolnavilor schizefreniai. Conferinta Nationala de Psihiatrie, Bucuresti, 1964.
12. P. BRINZEI: "Contribution a l'etude des exploations morphafonctionalles dans la Psychiatrie." *Ann. medico-psychol.*, 1, 1, 1964.
13. P. BRINZEI, M. SELERA, E. LAZAREANU, AND ST. RUSU: "Contributii la studiul dinemicei I[131] si p[32]." Conferinta Nationala de Psihiatrie, Bucuresti, 1964.
14. Coneluzile Consfatuirii privind, "Nevrosele." Bucuresti, Dec. 4–5, 1961. *Psih., Neur., Neurochir.*, 4, 293, 1962.
15. P. CORTEZ: Probleme de diagnostic in unele sindreame schizofrenoide. Conferinta Nationala de Psihiatrie, Bucuresti, 1964.
16. C. CSIKY: "Contributiuni la probleme etiopatogeniei schizofrenilar." Conferinta tinuta la Tg. Mu aprilie, 1960.
17. C. CSIKY: "Profilaxia bolilor psihice." *Neur., Psih., Neurochir.*, 2, 97, 1960.

18. C. CSIKY: "Consideretii asupre cadrului noxologic al diagnosticului si simptomatologiei schizofreniel." *Neur., Psih., Neurochir.*, 6, 1957.

19. C. CSIKY, P. KISE, R. CSIKY-WAGMER: Cerceta ri hemstalagice in schizofrenie. Conferinta Maticmala de Psihiatrie, 1964.

20. A. DESICS, SEN ALEX., VALENTINE NEICU, MARINA ROSCA, AND MARIE TOMERUG: "Tulburarile structurii legise a gindirii le schizofrenii stabilizeti." Conferinte Nationala de Psihistrie, Bucuresti, 1964.

21. AL. GALASESCU: Eforie Spitalelor civile din Bucuresti, 1900.

22. V. GEMEIU: "Istoria medicinei in Rominia," 1923.

23. C. HAMAUGIU: Cedul generel al Rominiei, vols. 2, 18.

24. I. IANCU, ELENA PAMPU: Contributii la studiul fisi opatolegic al schizofreniei la copil. "Probleme de Psihiatrie." Edit. Medicala, Bucuresti, 1957.

25. M. KERNBACH: *Miscares medicala romina*, 3, 7, 8, 162, 251, 1936.

26. N. MIHAESCU AND MARGARETE STEFAN: "Psihoprofilzxia starilor sechelare de limita, dupa leziunile cerebrale ale copilului." *Neur., Psih., Neurochir.*, 72, 1959.

27. I. MINCIU: Iacadres in cimpul muncii a bolnavilor psihiei remisi cu defect si a micilor mintali din reionul Cimpins, regiunee Ploesti. *Neur., Psih., Neurochir.*, 1958, p. 307, nr 4.

28. N. MINOVIC AND I. STANESCU: Conception nouvelle sur l-etialogie du crime. Volume Jubilaire en L'honeur du Prof. Dr. C. I. Parhon, Jassy, 1934.

29. N. NEICU AND I. STOICE: "Actiumes eserimed in epilepsia eu crize freevente." *Neur., Psih., Neurochir.* 1, 66, 1955.

30. R. RACALA, BALANESCU ST., AND C. CEATU: Citeve consideratiuni asupre personalitatii post-schizefrenice. Conferate Nationala de Psihistrie, Bucuresti, 1964.

31. E. PAMFIL: Responsebilitatee atenusti in expertize psihistriea. "Probleme de Psihiatries," Ed. Medicala, Bucuresti, 1957.

32. E. PAMFIL AND STASSEL ST.: "Alienstie schizofrenica si structurile logice." Conferinte Nationala de Psihiatrie, 1964.

33. C. I. PARHON: "Quelques mots sur les alienes criminals et les criminals alienes." Archives de Sociologie et Criminologie, 1916.

34. C. I. PARHON: Constitutia somato-psihica si raporturile en criminologia. *Bevite de dropt pomal si atiinta permitenciaral or.*, 3, 4, 9–10, 1930.

35. C. I. PARHON. Repertul dintre psihiatrie, atiinta dreptulni si criminolgie. *Reviate de dropt penal si stiinta pemitenciareler*, 8, 9, 1936.

36. C. I. PARHON, R. FELIX, AND E. SEMEN: Manifestari Psihopatalegice la batrini. "Probleme de psihistrie," Ed. Medicala, Bucuresti, 1957.

37. CONSTANTA PARHON-STEFANESCU, E. TOMERUG, AND M. CORTEZ: Contributiuni le studiul tulburarilor endocrine in sindroamale astenice. a les Conferinta de Neurologie, Psihiatrie si Neurochirurgie, Edit. Medicala, Bucaresti, 1955.

38. CONSTANTA PARHON-STEFANESCU, ELENA PREDA, AND FLORICA MEIU:

Contributiuni la studiul metaboliamului cerebral in report ou modificaeile mediului intern. *Bul. Acad. RPR, Sectia de Stiinte medicale*, vol. 7, 4, 1209, 1955.

39. CONSTANTA PARHON-STEFANESCU, ELENA PREDA, AND FLORICE MEIU: Contributii la studiul functiunii hepetice in schizofrenie. Iuerarile sesiunii stiintifice a Acad. C. I. Parhon, Iesi, 1957.

40. CONSTANTA PARHON-STEFANESCU, ELENA PREDA, FELICIA CHEREIMLESCU, AND FLORICA MEIU: "Contributiila studiul biologiei dementei senile." *Neur., Psih., Neurochir.* 1, 6, 1957.

41. CONSTANTA PARHON-STEFANESCU AND ILEANE VUJDEE: "Citeva cerebcetari cu privire la capacitates de munea a bolnavilor psihici." *Neur., Psih., Neurochir.*, 2, 156, 1957.

42. CONSTANTA PARHON-STEFANESCU, ALEXANDRINE RETEZEEMU, AND ILEANE VUJDEE: "Consideratii asupre incedrarii nosologice a schizofremille." *Neur., Psih., Neurochir.*, 3, 20, 1957.

43. CONSTANTA PARHON-STEFANESCU AND A. VREJAN: "Tireoidectomia kakmeted leconie affectivaih psihozev." *Jurn. neurol. i psih. im SS Kersakova*, 8, 1005, 1957.

44. CONSTANTA PARHON-STEFANESCU, ELENA PREDA, AND FLORICA MEIU: "Nei cercetari asupre biologice dementei senile." *Neur., Psih, Neurochir.*, 3, 265, 1958.

45. CONSTANTA PARHON-STEFANESCU, ELENA PREDA, AND FLORICA MEIU: "Consideratii asupre tulburarilor exidative in sindromul schizofrenic." *Neur., Psih., Neurochir.*, 2, 107, 1958.

46. CONSTANTA PARHON-STEFANESCU: "Psihistrie sterceskci vozreste," *Nevropet. i psih. im Korsakova*, 11, 1257, 1959.

47. CONSTANTA PARHON-STEFANESCU AND Z. RODIN: "Episod psihotic paranoid aparut in cursul unei hipertiroidii," *Neur., Psih., Neurochir.*, 6, 481, 1959.

48. CONSTANTA PARHON-STEFANESCU: "Consideratii asupre cadrulu Diagnosticului Nevrosei Astenice." *Neur., Psih., Neurochir.*, 14, 293, 1962.

49. CONSTANTA PARHON-STEFANESCU, Z. RODIN, AND ARSENE AURORA: "Consideration sur la fonction du cortex surrenal dans les malades psychiques," *Ann. Medico-psychologique*, vol. 11, 2, 181, 1963.

50. CONSTANTA PARHON-STEFANESCU, AND E. TOMERUG: Uber strafberem Handlungen des Arteriosclerosekreaken. Kulanlenyomat idegrendozer verkeringesenek elettana es klininikuma psichopharmakologi Klinikai vonatkozasar, Debrecem 219, 1964.

51. CONSTANTA PARHON-STEFANESCU AND I. CANTACUZINO: Evolution et orientation de le psychiatrie roumaine. Communication presentee au XIX-e Congres International d'Historie de la Medecine. Bale, 7–12, Septembre 1964.

52. CONSTANTA PARHON-STEFANESCU AND AL. SEN. MARINA ROSC: "Unele aspecte ale eficiemtei perceptiei in starile astemice si depresive." *Neur., Psih., Neurochir.*, 1, 2, 1964.

53. T. PIROZYNSKI ST GH. SCRIPCRU: "Consideratii generale asupre criteriilor de responsabilitate a bolmevil or psihici." *Neur., Psih., Neurochir.*, 3, 261, 1963.

54. CH. PREDA: "Citeva consideretiuni asupre moilor conceptii de igiena si prefilazie neuropsihica." *Neur., Psih., Neurochir.*, 4, 75, 1956.

55. V. PREDESCU: "Diagnestical ai perticularitatile clinice ale umer psihose halucinator-delirante de natura arteriosclerotica." *Neur., Psih., Neurochir.*, 4, 297, 1961.

56. V. PREDESCU, I. REMAN, E. PARESCHIVESCU, K. CRISTIAN, D. KRILAVIET, ST. PIREE, V. MIRONTOV, L. VIA, M. BRESLA, AND P. BENGULESCU: Contributii la studiul electroencefalografic si pneumonencefalegrefic al bolnavilor de schizofrenie in diversale stadif de evolutie a belii. Conferinta Nationala de Psihiatrie, 1964.

57. ALEXANDRINE RETEZEANU, E. TOMERUG, AND S. ELIAS: "Psihosa periodiea le o hipertiroidiana in ti sareinei." *Neur., Psih., Neurochir.*, 4, 305, 1960.

58. ALEXANDRINE RETEZEANU, S. ELIAS, AND D. CIOBAMU: "Tulburari psihice in curcul decompensarilor cardiace." *Neur., Psih., Neurochir.*, 1, 45, 1961.

59. P. SAMRIEN: Medicine si farmacia in trecutul rominesc.

60. Monitorul medical al Principatelor Unite, 14, 1864.

61. M. SERBEN, D. ALEX C. WOLFSHAUT, AND A. AARU: Tulburari ale functiei overiene in nevroza. A. 18-e Conferinta de Neurologie, Psthietrie si Neurchirurgie, Editure medicala, Bucuresti, 1955.

62. GH. SIMIONESCU: Orientari actuale in practica expertized psihistrico-judiciare in Republiea Populara Romina. *Neur., Psih., Neurochir.*, 2, 1963.

63. E. TOMERUG: Notiuni de psihistrie judiciara, Bucuresti, 1957.

64. E. TOMERUG: Schizophrenie und Kriminalitat. II Kengres International des Psichiatrie, Zurich, vol. 4, 1957–1959.

65. E. TOMERUG: "Problems psihiatriei judiciare in R.P.R. Prebleme de psihiatrie," Ed. Medicala, Bucresti, 1957.

66. E. TOMERUG, N. DISCONESCU, I. GOLUMBEAM, AND S. SERBANESCU: "Responsebilitates minorilor care comit acte infractionale." *Neur., Psih., Neurochir.*, 5, 465, 1963.

67. E. TOMERUG, N. DISCONESCU, AND E. UNGUREANU: Particularitatile medico-legale intilnite de balnevi de schizofrenie in functie de ferme clinica a bolii. Conferinta metinala de Psihiatrie, Bucresti, 1964.

68. N. VASILESCU: Asupre interpretarii greaite a notiunii de ne vrexa in practice medicali. A 18- Conferinta de Neurologie, Psihiatrie si Neurochirurgie, Edit. Medicela, Bucuresti, 1955.

69. C. A. WOLFSHAUT, INPULESEU, AND I. TRIFAN: Nevrose eu simptome endocrine. A 18-a Conferinta de Neurologie, Psihiatrie si Neurologie, Editure Medicala, Bucuresti, 1955.

CHAPTER TEN

Mental Health in China

BY
DR. GREGORIO BERMANN

HISTORY OF CHINESE PSYCHIATRY

THE HISTORY OF PSYCHIATRY IN CHINA may be divided into three periods: (a) to the end of the last century; (b) the foreign period, beginning with the founding of the first psychiatric hospital; (c) since the Liberation.

To the End of the Last Century

The first written testimony concerning mental illnesses dates from the fourteenth century B.C. The act of attributing headaches to the wind which sweeps the valleys of the Yellow River is recorded in the *bone oracles* of that period. From that time on there are numerous texts which refer to nervous and mental diseases and to their treatment. The importance accorded to those diseases is evident from the fact that when the Imperial College of Medicine was established in 1060 A.D., 30 of the 120 students were to dedicate themselves in a special department to the knowledge of such ailments, referred to as "illnesses of the wind." During a previous period, Ch'ao Iuangfang, in the year 610, in the *General Treatise on the Causes and Symptoms of Diseases,* describes no less than fifty-nine nervous and mental diseases, from hysteria and apoplexy to speech disorders and facial paralysis. Wang K'en-tang in 1608 (during the Ming dynasty) classified psychiatric illnesses into three groups: alienation—in which schizophrenia is noted—madness, and fits.

The insane person is sometimes violent, sometimes stupid, singing and laughing or sad and weeping. He gets no better even after months and years. The common name for this disorder is wind in the mind. Those with frustrated ambitions are liable to be so affected.

The patient is boisterous, garrulous, raving, stubborn and violent. He abuses everyone indiscriminately—friends, relatives and strangers. He may even climb any eminence at hand, sing at the top of his voice, take off his clothes and run away, climbing over the wall or onto the roof in a way that no normal person would be able to do. He may tell of things that were never seen.

The person subject to fits becomes dizzy and cannot recognize people. He falls to the ground, having convulsions and suffering from jerks over which he has no control.

The treatments varied according to the medical school and their theories of diseases; they included the uses of numerous herbs, drugs of animal and mineral origin, and certainly acupuncture and superficial cauterization. Superstition, animistic beliefs, and assurances of demoniacal possession or divine punishment were widespread as were practices of magic, spells, enchantments, and exorcisms. In the history of ancient Chinese medicine there is found a singular mixture of quackery and charlatanism, which nevertheless aspired to redeem itself through its valid aspects. Frequently, its practitioners were not highly regarded. In the T'ang annals one reads: "Mathematicians, land surveyors, fortune tellers, physiognomists, physicians, and necromancers were charlatans. The learned did not consider them to be well-informed people."

The insane were left in the care of their relatives; they wandered from one place to another, and when they became dangerous and bothersome, they were locked up in cells, subject to chaining.

The Foreign Period

The first attempt to establish a psychiatric institution dates back to the end of the last century. Although it had been suggested in 1874, Dr. John Kerr was not able to establish such an institution in Canton until

1897, with an endowment of thirty beds. It grew rapidly until it held 500 places; it was arbitrarily closed in 1937 because of labor unrest. During the thirty years until 1927, 6,599 patients were admitted, and of these 27 percent were cured. It is said that prior to this hospital in Canton, there were two small centers in China: the Chinese Insane Asylum in Faitham, opened in 1885, and another in Hong Kong. Neither of these took long in disappearing. The first mention of a psychiatry course at the College of Medicine in Hong Kong dates back to 1905. In Canton, Dr. A. H. Woods taught regular courses in neurology and psychiatry beginning in 1910. In 1919 he moved to the Peking Union Medical College where he again taught these specialties. In Peking, there existed since 1906 a small psychiatric asylum adjoining the Municipal Hospital. In 1933, the Department of Social Welfare, in collaboration with the Peking Union Medical College, reorganized and transformed it into the Peking City Psychopathic Hospital with a 200-bed capacity. The Peking group carried out scientific tasks and in 1939 published its results in *Social and Psychological Studies in Neuropsychiatry in China*.

The most valuable work during that period was accomplished in Shanghai. Shanghai was in 1931 the most populated Chinese city, with three million inhabitants, and it grew, particularly through the influx of refugees, until in 1937 it held approximately five million people. In 1931, Dr. R. S. Lyman, a graduate of the Johns Hopkins University School of Medicine, initiated classes in neurology and psychiatry; he was succeeded in the following year by Dr. Barrie. The most important contribution in terms of assistance and prevention came from Dr. Fanny G. Halpern, who had been a teacher at the University of Vienna. In 1934, she began the teaching of neurology and psychiatry and organized a neurology section in the first hospital of the Red Cross Society of China; she also undertook the training of psychiatric nurses. The National Medical College, the Medical School of St. John's University, and the Women's Christian Medical College of Shanghai jointly shared her teaching. In June, 1935, the Mercy Hospital for Nervous Diseases was opened with 600 beds and eleven buildings; this institution became the center of instruction for the specialty. The Foreign Mission Sisters of St. Dominic of Mary Knoll and the Brothers of Charity from Trier, Germany, constituted the nursing staff. Dr. Halpern organized study groups and held numerous conferences with charitable organizations to promote scientific methods of treatment and the launching of a prophylaxis campaign. She formed a committee to consider legislation about the insane; however, the Sino-Japanese war, which began in 1937, blocked the development of her ambitious program. In June, 1944, during the Japanese occupation, Dr. Halpern's activities ceased. When the war terminated in 1945, a few attempts were made to resume previous tasks, but because of the departure of many trained staff members, these attempts were frustrated.

In a speech delivered in May, 1938, Dr. R. Wang indicated what had been accomplished up to that time:

As a Chinese physician, I wish to give you a bird's-eye view of what has already been accomplished . . . (1) Five years ago, in all East and Central China there was not a single medical or nursing school where a regular course of treatment for mental and nervous disease was given. (2) The institutions for the mentally ill were still of the asylum type. (3) Simply nothing of preventive work in psychiatry or (4) about legal Codes concerning mental patients, existed. . . . Today, (1) we have . . . courses in neurology and psychiatry . . . in the Shanghai medical colleges. (2) Some Chinese physicians are now interested in specializing in this line, and (3) a modern mental hospital (Mercy) has been established . . . Five years ago, on Dr. Halpern's arrival in China, (4) no staff was available to assist her in clinical work; but now we have a staff of well-trained Chinese physicians and nurses, graduated in successive years. . . . (5) We have introduced the most modern, scientific therapy—the same as that used in other modern countries. (6) Educational campaigns of four years past have taught the Chinese the necessity of sending the insane patients to mental institutions, where formerly they were either left in chains at home, among nursing mothers and little children, or sent to Buddhist monks, to live in their temples—or elsewhere to one of their 101 sects. (7) Another advance is that Chinese physicians now frequently request consultations with psychiatrists. . . . (8) A child guidance clinic in our division at the Red Cross Hospital was recently taken in charge by us psychiatrists from the National Medical College.

Most mental hygiene activities, such as the expansion of the Committee on Mental Welfare of the Club Institute, were initiated in Shanghai. The first mental hygiene clinic, directed by Dr. Halpern, was opened in January, 1940, at St. John's University Medical School. Dr. Charles Hart Westbrook took charge of psychology and mental tests. He presided over the Mental Hygiene Association of Shanghai, which was reorganized in May, 1940, and was still functioning at the end of 1953. A branch of the Mental Hygiene Association was founded in 1948 in Chungking.

Similar activities were also begun in other parts of China. At the Central University of Nanking, Dr. Chen Yui Long taught the first course in psychiatry; soon, however, because of the capture of the city by the Japanese, he had to stop his instruction. After his evacuation to Chengtu,

Dr. Chen continued his teaching at the West China Union University, where he established a psychiatric hospital and a child behavior clinic.

The descriptions of psychiatric-aid facilities give little indication of the primitive conditions. The statistics relating to the number of insane are not well founded. It was customarily believed that there were fewer insane in China than in other countries because of the quiet life and the lack of preoccupation with daily problems, in contrast with the conflicts and growing tensions in the West. In truth, this was not so. A 1912 report from the Kerr Memorial Hospital of Canton states: "We are forced to conclude that insanity is as common, if not more common, than in the West." In 1930, Drs. I. S. Wang and M. P. Yung stated that "It is our opinion that insanity is as common in China as in Europe and in the United States." In 1926, Dr. L. J. Harvey estimated that there was 1 insane per each 1,000 of population, which would have meant at that time some 400,000 mentally ill. In an editorial appearing in the same issue of the Chinese Medical Journal, it was estimated that the ratio was 1 per 400, which would have meant from 1,000,000 to 1,250,000 insane, inasmuch as there were from 400 to 500 million inhabitants. Dr. J. L. McCartney, who was born and practiced psychiatry in China, calculated in 1927 (following extensive investigations by means of questionnaires) that there were 3,120,000 nervous and mental cases, 1,140,000 requiring hospitalization, and that 1 of 126 among the ill was a neuropsychiatric case.

In 1947, Professor Karl M. Bowman was sent to China by the World Health Organization of the United Nations to help found the National Neuropsychiatric Institute. He arrived in Nanking, capital of Nationalist China, in August of that year, and stayed there three months gathering facts. On May 20, 1948, he presented the results of his observations to the Annual Congress of the American Psychiatric Association. He submitted evidence that China, with more than 450 million inhabitants had fewer than 6,000 beds for the mentally ill*; that it had less than fifty psychiatrists; that of the fifty medical schools, only a few offered discrete instruction in psychiatry; and that there was no possibility of contracting with professors inasmuch as there was no money with

---

* The data varies from one traveler to another. Thus, Academician Popov of Moscow writes that in 1949 there were only four psychiatric hospitals in Peking, Shanghai, Canton, and Nanking, with a total of 1,000 beds and not more than sixty psychiatrists.

which to pay them. Bowman was under the impression that the mental diseases were essentially the same as in the United States. He found no supporting reasons to show that the Chinese differ fundamentally from any other races. The idea, for example, that the Chinese are phlegmatic, cold, and foolish does not stand up under observation. Bowman recognized that many changes have taken place in Chinese culture and customs, quite a few of which originated in the United States. There is a rupture, or at least an estrangement, from traditional customs and habits. He declared that the newly developing attitudes are of the greatest importance: "There is a great danger that its culture will adopt many of the American features and abandon some of the best of the old Chinese culture. Thus, for example, the emotional family atmosphere which is healthier, perhaps because the Chinese mother displays less neurotic concern for her children, is bound to change, leading to a neurotic attitude similar to that of the North American mother. For this reason, one considers that the development of psychiatry in China, together with an educational effort in mental hygiene, can offer something very important and have a profound effect upon the entire cultural attitude during the next century."

Perhaps the most generally known psychiatric problem, and at the same time the one symptomatic of China's mental deterioration, was the spread of addiction to opium and to other toxic agents. Although opium smoking had begun in the seventeenth century, as early as 1729 the emperor Yung Chen issued the first decree against its trade. After 1840, the Opium Wars contributed enormously toward its dissemination. The drastic decrees, some of which dealt harshly—including the death penalty—with opium contraband, were of little value. Without embargo, the international and national campaigns, and above all those of the League of Nations, against its commerce contributed to a decrease in its production. Indeed, in 1934, 5,856 tons of opium were produced; by 1937, production had decreased to 891 tons. Of the 18,500 tons sold during these four years, 1,350 (7.1 percent) were employed for medical use, and the remainder, a great part of which was consumed in China, was used by addicts. Thereafter, during the occupation, the Japanese undertook to increase its use, to debilitate the Chinese physically and morally. The greatest portion of the opium was smoked, some was chewed, and some taken in liquid form or through injections. Its euphoric effects, with an erotic coloration, are known. The number of addicts is not known. In 1935, T. Pai set 300,000 as an approximate estimate of the number of addicts in the Peking zone. If one takes into account that the population numbered 1,500,000, this means one addict per each five persons! During that period 3,768,308 opium addicts had registered in sixteen of the twenty-eight provinces and municipalities. Z. Klan, based on a review of world literature, asserts that the opium smokers in China climbed to the enormous total of forty million. Knud O. Moller pointed out that other addictions were also widespread; thus in the year 1932, at least five tons of heroin per month were introduced through three Chinese ports, while the world medical needs for heroin amounted to hardly one ton.

Since the Liberation

Present psychiatric assistance must be considered within the context of the social situation and within the framework of health. The inheritance which the ruling regime received was laden with terrible burdens, devastating epidemics, an undernourished population with a standard of living low in all its aspects, natural calamities which had not been properly confronted, a very poor standard of sanitation, anarchy in welfare, and ignorance and superstitions. Even when there were no valid statistics, it was calculated that there were approximately 30 deaths per thousand annually, of which half were avoidable, or, in other words, 7.5 million for a population of 500 million. Of these figures, some 20 percent occurred in beings less than 1 year old, at the rate of 200 to 250 per 1,000 births, the majority of these deaths due to gastrointestinal diseases. Of the other cases of excess deaths, approximately 1 million were attributable to tuberculosis and an equal number to smallpox. In 1927, the Peking Public Health Station stated that 39.4 percent died without any medical attention, 44.3 percent were attended by traditional physicians, and only 16.3 percent by modern doctors. In one of the best factories of North China, 95 percent of those employed on the premises suffered from trachoma, and more than half displayed symptoms of undernourishment. In another study, covering 1,200 students in 5 schools, 14.1 percent had trachoma, 16.2 percent infected tonsils, 30.9 percent dental caries.[14]

On the other hand, there was great inequality in development and sanitary conditions in different parts of the country. Whereas there were provinces, in particular, the coastal provinces, with more than 200 inhabitants per square kilometer, there were others, such as Sinkiang or the autonomous region of Tibet, with 1 to 5 inhabitants per square kilometer, also almost without doctors, and Shanghai had 1 physician per each 1,000 inhabitants. In vast rural areas, attention to sanitation was very deficient, dependent upon herbmen, untrained midwives, and even sorcerers. In Shanghai, the most modern of cities, with the majority of the midwives, some 30 percent of the deliveries took place without any medical help. At the time of the liberation in 1949, the renowned city of Peking accumulated more than 200,000 tons of refuse and garbage which were cleaned up by 73,000 volunteers who used 36,000 vehicles. In all China in 1949 there were 90,000 hospital beds for more than 500 million inhabitants. During the previous forty years, less than 20,000 doctors, 300 odontologists, 2,000 pharmacists, 13,000 nurses and 10,000 obstetricians were graduated from its medical schools; there were also half a million old-fashioned doctors practicing medicine.

The program established by the government in 1949 adhered to these five principles: (a) The health of the population is the responsibility of the government; (b) agrarian reform and industrial organization will increase the standard of living, which is the most important and essential basis for any sanitary work; (c) the work of the masses of the population is in the glorious tradition of revolutionary humanitarianism; (d) the most advanced sanitary principles will be utilized, with the example and help of the U.S.S.R.; (e) advances must be achieved through the active participation of each member of the great masses. The first National Sanitation Conference which was held in Peking in August, 1950, unanimously adopted these guiding principles for the sanitation tasks of New China: All sanitation work must be directed toward serving the people, centering the greatest attention upon the workers, peasants, and soldiers; prophylactic medicine must be emphasized; and the closest coordination must be established between modern and old-fashioned doctors. As was stated by the nation's Public Health Minister, Li Teh-chuan, the country prepared itself to provide the necessary five million hospital beds, to train half a million doctors and three to four million auxiliary medical personnel.

It was thus understood that the authorities would favor these great problems with their attention and that psychiatric assistance would occupy a secondary place. As has been repeatedly stated, psychiatry constituted the weakest link in Chinese medicine. With all this, the nervous and mentally ill were not neglected. As early as 1957, there were nineteen times more psychiatric beds than in 1949, with a large number of second rank, more or less qualified, but undeniably devoted health personnel.

As was pointed out by Feng Ying-k'un, during the thirty years preceding the Liberation there had not been more than 200 neurological and psychiatric articles and two books published, whereas in the subsequent years there were many more than during the previous period. One can follow the growing development of the specialization in the *Chinese Neurological and Psychiatric Journal*, which is published every two months as the organ of the Chinese Society of Neurology and Psychiatry, founded in 1952. Its text is in Chinese, but the principal articles contain English resumes. Numerous articles on psychiatry have also been published in the English language *Chinese Medical Journal*. Since 1964 the Chinese Academy has published a journal in English with resumes of the principal articles from the medical journals in the country. Some of the articles in the *Chinese Neurological and Psychiatric Journal* are summarized in the German Democratic Republic's *Die Medizin der Sowjetunion und der Volksdemokratien im Referat*.

TRADITIONAL CHINESE MEDICINE AND PSYCHIATRY

Hundreds of thousands of physicians practice traditional medicine in China. In 1965, a Vice-Minister of Public Health cited a figure of 350,000. At present, at the advanced as well as at the intermediate level, eighteen of the ninety medical schools are dedicated to traditional medicine. The Peking School in 1957 consisted of five departments: internal medicine, surgery, acupuncture and cauterization, pharmacy and the study of herbs and the history of national medicine.

In China, research is not limited by Western standards of empiricism; leaves and roots are being analyzed in order to compare their effectiveness and to transform them into pills and other convenient medicinal forms. Gymnastic methods—in particular, the special psychological respiratory gymnastics—are considered valuable. The Chinese are famed as masseurs. They are also well versed in hygienic and dietetic precepts. Acupuncture and moxibustion are dynamic treatments of the states of inhibition to reduce physical as well as psychic pain. Their stimulation of moderate and prolonged reflexes which act upon the internal organs and the cerebral cortex is in accordance with Pavlov's stressing of the propagation of negative inducement, or of the inhibition of the cortical regions toward the peripheral elements. As he wrote: "The fact that each point on the skin is protected by a corresponding point in the cerebral cortex demonstrates clearly the advantage offered in physiology by cutaneous analysors for the study of the processes of inhibition, inasmuch as the cutaneous analysors are accessible on the entire surface of the skin."

I was informed by the director of the institute in Hopei Province that these traditional methods, applied to psychoses, achieve results superior to those obtained with insulin and electroshock therapy. With acupuncture, Hwang Sin-lin states that he has achieved 99 percent success in the treatment of violent headaches; Wang Ching-pu and his collaborators are satisfied with this method in the case of neurotic symptoms; Cerny states that in Si An there is an interest in electropuncture and that special apparatus has been designed for this purpose.*

The therapeutic results obtained in the six Chinese national establishments, from September, 1951, to the end of December, 1952, are given in the following table:†

Illness	Number of Cases	Cures	Appre-ciable improve-ment	Partial improve-ment	No Change
Headaches	407	188	111	90	18
Migraines	39	19	7	11	2
Poliomyelitis (with period of paralysis)	37		15	16	6
Neuralgia, sciatica	119	52	29	32	6
Neuralgia (trigeminal)	54	28	9	15	2
Chronic rheumatism	2,169	768	681	604	116
Traumatic arthritis	37	23	6	7	1
Rheumatoid arthritis	37	8	8	17	4
Pulmonary tuberculosis	35	8	10	9	8
Constipation	84	54	19	11	8
Malaria	23	23			

† Data from the French journal *Horizons*, May, 1958.

* Claude Le Brestre mentions some equipment developed and used in France— the European country where acupuncture has perhaps been employed first and to the largest extent—namely, the electroprobe and De La Fuye implanted needle, the Brunet-Gremr measuring probe, the Walter "Ultratone," and the Martiny sound probe.

PSYCHIATRIC TREATMENT

Since the communists came to power, psychiatric treatment has undergone noticeable development. At first, existing health institutions were utilized without immediate reorganization. Subsequently, these institutions were enlarged, and new ones were created. Numerous hospitals and clinics were established in regions that had until then been almost totally deprived of psychiatric services. On the occasion of the tenth anniversary of the Revolution (1959), various authors celebrated the results achieved. These articles state that 62 new psychiatric hospitals, with a number of beds 14 times greater than that before the Liberation—although no numbers are mentioned—were built in 21 provinces and autonomous regions. In 1950 the psychiatric beds numbered 1.1 percent of the total number of hospital beds; in 1957, 3.6 percent. In 1958, the number of doctors in psychiatric hospitals was 16 times greater than in 1949, and the number of patients increased more than 20 times. Psychiatrists of superior and average caliber were rapidly trained in different medical schools; 375 were trained in Shanghai and Nanking between 1953 and 1958. Thanks to the methods of treatment, the percentage of improvement, which was 50 percent in 1950, rose to 80 percent in 1958.*

The history of the Shanghai Municipal Psychiatric Hospital demonstrates the changes which have taken place. Before the founding of the institution in 1934, many of the insane wandered through the streets of Shanghai, were confined to their homes, or were locked up in gloomy police quarters.

The hospital was constructed with resources supplied in equal parts by the Kuomintang and private donations. The total of 200 beds were divided among four wards. The first was extremely luxurious, had forty to fifty beds, and drew a monthly fee of $1,500 from each occupant. It was almost entirely vacant, so that it was subsequently transformed into quarters for the personnel. A patient in the second ward paid from $500 to $1,000 per month; the third and fourth wards were for charity and

---

* Unfortunately, the information which we were able to gather is insufficient and fragmentary because the psychiatric facilities are in the hands of regional, provincial, or municipal authorities, and frequently within the same province or city the activities of neighbors are ignored as if they were in watertight compartments. The Chinese Ministry of Health lacks a central agency, a type of national institute of mental health, to centralize psychiatric treatment, and consequently it cannot supply information in this regard. Most of the facts assembled here were gathered personally by the author during his visits to four major cities.

were constantly overcrowded. In these last, 30 percent died annually, so that the hospital had a bad reputation. A doctor visited twice weekly. Sometimes there was no more than one nurse, and the methods of treatment were very primitive. From 1949 to 1952 the system deteriorated steadily; this provoked complaints and protests which in 1952 caused the intervention and the take-over of the establishment by the State. However, the same management continued until 1954, at which time it was eliminated because of the discovery of conspiratorial activities.

After the assumption of control by the State, beds were increased from 200 to 2,500*, with adequate budget and personnel. The administration, or rather the judgment of the nuns who served it, was regulated, and it was separated from the clinical and scientific management. The conduct of the personnel toward the patients changed radically: Isolation, confinement, punishment, and repression were abolished. It was decided that the personnel should live, eat, and even sleep together in friendship and solidarity with the patients. After four years of this new treatment of the majority of patients, forty-four of the worst cases with more than fifteen years hospitalization, among whom more than 70 percent exhibited destructive psychoses, were chosen to be treated by these new methods. The results were very encouraging: Four were discharged, four worked well, many others looked after their personal cleanliness and participated in community life. In the beginning, twenty-five male nurses and servants were assigned to the forty-four patients. Now fifteen watch over seventy. The wards are now regulated, the sick are clean, they are not destructive or aggressive, and community life is smooth and productive.

Mental health cannot depend solely on the attention paid by doctors; the patient's mind should be as active as possible. Patients are taken to public displays, for walks and to shows. News in the daily newspapers, on radio or on TV is explained. Naturally, there is also much room in this program for different types of work, be it domestic or semi-industrial, and for recreation (singing, choruses, dances, etc.). The activities should be varied: If life is monotonous, the patients will not improve and may relapse. Modern treatments, as well as traditional medicine are used whenever necessary. Of most importance, however, is the conviction of the personnel that patients worsen when they are submerged in their own pathological thoughts, which contribute to their isolation from society.

Together with Professor Hsuh, I visited a psychiatric hospital some

---

* In 1957 during my first visit to Shanghai, psychiatric beds numbered 900, attended by 60 specialists; in 1965 there were 2,500, with 90 psychiatrists.

twenty kilometers from Shanghai. It has room for 460 patients and employs a total of 420, of which 64 are psychiatrists, 261 nurses (8 chief nurses and 66 nurses' aides), and 60 administrative employees. Each nurse receives 60 yens per month ($25). The average confinement is 86 days. Cures and remissions exceed 80 percent.

The psychiatric needs of Peking are served by four principal establishments, one for acute cases and three for chronic cases. The first had 420 beds in 1965. Of the 330 personnel, 224 were medically trained and of these 34 were doctors. On the average, 140 new patients are admitted monthly. The hospital is adequately organized, with a laboratory, occupational therapy services, recreational activities, and a nutritious diet.

In Kwantung Province, psychiatric interest was concentrated in the capital, Canton. The university's psychiatric hospital, under the direction of Dr. Mo Kan-ming, has 600 beds in well-furnished wards and is equipped with biology, biochemistry, and anatomy-pathology laboratories. Service is provided by 400 persons—9 times more than in 1949—and of these 58 are doctors and more than 200 are nurses. The psychiatrists were trained in Canton proper. In addition, there are in the province a 600-bed colony for chronic cases, two mobile units (one of which is in the city), and a few other services in keeping with the local needs. Boarding expenses are covered by the communal authorities and by the patients' families.

The Psychiatric Hospital of Nanking is municipal. It has 400 beds and the only department of child psychiatry in China, with twenty-four patients.

There are other establishments and mobile units in other provinces and regions. Cerny advises that in Umurruchi, capital of the autonomous region of Sinkiang-Uighur in the northwest, three psychiatrists are working as part of the health-center program.

During the period of economic recovery (1949–1952) the proportion of psychiatric admissions in relation to the total numbers in the hospitals was 6.8 percent; from 1952 to 1957, 21 percent; and from 1958 to 1965, 12 percent. In general, the psychiatric hospitals and services in China which I visited do not differ significantly from those in the West.

SOME ILLNESSES AND THEIR TREATMENT

In José Itzigsohn's statistics of 1956, dealing with admissions during the previous six years to the Clinic of the Department of Psychiatry of Peking (sixty beds), to which acute cases are preferably admitted, this is the number of the psychoses and neuroses:

Psychoses	*Number*
Schizophrenia	
Paranoid form	154
Catatonic form	44
Hebephrenic form	22
Simple form	11
Unclassified	44
Manic-depressive Psychoses	
Manics	50
Depressives	26
Involute Psychosis	
Paranoids	9
Depressives	6
Traumatic psychosis	13
Hypertensive psychoses	13
Syphilitics	9
Infectious psychoses	12
Toxic psychoses	12
Psychoses caused by medicinal intoxication	8
Psychoses caused by gas	2
Psychoses suspected to be caused by alcoholism	2
Epileptic psychosis	4
Reactive psychoses	20
Cerebral arteriosclerosis	3
Oligophrenia	1
Alzheimer sickness	1
Neuroses	
Neurasthenia	107
Hysteria	48
Obsessive Neurosis	8
Psychoasthenia	3
Psychopathic personalities	6
Unclassified	8

Schizophrenia

As in the West, the schizophrenia group is the most important psychiatric problem. During a 21-year period, statistics from Shanghai point to 3,329 schizophrenics out of 4,506 psychoses. Hsia-Chen-yi selected 2,000 schizophrenics out of this group and obtained the following figures: 1.3 percent were under 15 years old; 50 percent were between 21 and 30 years old; over 7 percent were more than 40 years old; there were no differences with regard to sex. Insofar as reference is made to etiological factors, 70 percent consisted of a type lacking in superior nervous activity, 54 percent exhibited notorious psychic trauma, 9.7 percent infections and other somatic disease, 22 percent had family antecedents with mental illnesses. The paranoid form was dominant (46 percent), 15 percent were hebephrenics, 11 percent catatonics, 24 percent unclassified (the percentage of the simple form is not mentioned). Insulin shock, cardiazole, occupational therapy and psychotherapy were employed with these 2,000 patients.

In a study of schizophrenia by Drs. Hsa, T'ao, and Wang, 48 percent displayed the paranoid form, 16.5 percent were sexual maniacs, 11.4 percent were of the excited type, 2.8 percent of the simple form, 21.3 percent of other types. In this same study the chosen treatment was insulin shock, which was applied on a large scale in the Nanking Hospital. One of the treatments which proved to be effective was hydergin at an average dose of from 100 to 400 mg. The best results were obtained with the excited forms, thereafter with the paranoid forms, and the worst with the simple schizophrenias. The results depended also upon the duration of the illness. When less than 6 months, the cures and remissions rose to 82 percent; 50 percent if the duration was between 1 and 2 years; and 26 percent if the duration was more than 5 years.

Naturally investigations of the nature of the illness have been carried out. Using the acetyaldehyde test on 172 schizophrenics, in comparison with 158 psychopathics of other types and 58 neuropathics, Chi Ming proved that schizophrenics had more difficulty in digesting amino acids. Electroencephalographic studies are numerous. In an investigation performed at the Shanghai Municipal Mental Hospital, the results obtained with sugar, wheat flour, and roasted rice in ending the insulin coma were compared and the good results obtained with rice were demonstrated; with this cereal, none of the patients was nauseous, vomited, had diarrhea, or had prolonged comas, as was frequently the case with the other groups of patients; the authors believe that these good results are due to the fact that the gastrointestinal tract of a Chinese patient is more accustomed to rice than to sugar or to wheat flour.[10] If the scarcity of glucose caused them to attempt the termination of the coma with these products, the lack of insulin obliged them to reduce its consumption in the refractory cases, using 0.5 mg. injections of pilocarpine for the purpose.

Manic-depressive Psychoses

Attention is called to the limited number of depressions, particularly in view of the social upheavals to which the Chinese were subjected. Similar situations in other countries yielded higher percentages. Reactive psychoses are also diagnosed infrequently.

The best results against manic-depressive psychoses have been obtained with the convulsive treatment. In the cases of mania, Prof. U-chen-i of Peking was satisfied with the use, if necessary, of hypoglucemic shock, with comas of up to fifteen minutes' duration, obtaining 100 percent cures. Psychopharmacologically prolonged sleep and balneotherapy are also employed.

Psychiatry of Old Age

In China, old people are not a problem. The family, which formerly was weakened in its ties, is today strengthened. Rejection of those who because of their age cannot contribute financially does not exist. Children feel and practice the primordial duty of attending to and supporting their parents, the more so if these are invalids. Veneration of and obedience to the aged, pillars of ancient Chinese morality, are today perhaps greater than they were a few decades ago. If the aged do not have a family, they are cared for under favorable conditions in "institutions for the aged." In addition to that which they may receive for their minor expenses, they can always count upon the five securities: food, clothing, fuel, instruction for their children, burial.

Although they are exempt from duty, the aged continue to render services within their ability, mostly by caring for children while the parents are busy at work.

If the emotional life of the old ones is satisfied—and it is well known how much the needs for affection and solicitude count in the genesis of their pathology—their physical care does not count any less. It has been demonstrated that the aged formerly suffered from undernourishment and so many infectious diseases that frequently they terminated their own lives; they are given adequate medical care and they eat in conformity with their needs.

Mental Pathology of Circulatory Origin

Although arteriosclerosis and cerebral hypertension appear to occur to a greater degree than was supposed, it seems that their occurrence is less than in the West (partly because the average Chinese lifespan is shorter.) In a recent unpublished thesis, of 438 cases of insanity in the University Hospital of Peking, 9 were due to hypertensive diseases, only 2 to arteriosclerosis.

It is possible that the diet of rice and other vegetables and the limited use of butter and milk are partly responsible for these small numbers. On the other hand, the life of the peasants who form the immense majority of the population would not be greatly exposed to the psychic tensions which probably contribute to arthero and arteriosclerosis; however, as pointed out by Itzigsohn, foreign invasions and revolutionary wars, which during the last century stirred the country from one extremity to the other, made life difficult and painful.

Alcoholism and Toxicomanias

The consumption of wines and white beverages is limited, and cases of alcoholism are very few. Alcoholism is not the great problem in China that it is in other countries. In Shanghai, I was informed that since 1938 only three cases of delirium tremens had been noted, and two of these were in foreigners. In the aforementioned Peking statistics, only two cases of suspected alcoholism in six years are mentioned.

The problem of opium and other toxicomanias, which had been of such extraordinary magnitude, diminished in scope shortly after 1949. From that time on the new regime, which took drastic and definitive means, stopped the traffic in opium and other toxicomanic drugs. Jan Cerny compares the present situation with that of the British colony of Hong Kong: In 1959, with three million inhabitants, almost all Chinese, it was estimated (according to 1962 figures from the World Health Organization) that the number of toxicomaniacs there ranged between 150,000 and 200,000.

Psychopathic Personalities

The tendency in China of attributing abnormal conduct to social factors and errors and to the formulation and education of persons, rather than to endogenous causes, is notorious. Professor Hsa of Shanghai attributes the extreme rarity of psychopaths to the educational system in China. In the midst of a good family and social life, problems of conduct among children are few, although they sometimes exist in families with only one child or in those of former capitalists. Statistics (which do not include former capitalists) from the Clinic of the University of Peking mention 6 cases of psychopathic personality among 612 psychotic and neurotic patients admitted between 1949 and 1955. During the visits which I made to prisons (where there are many psychopaths in Western countries) its existence was not mentioned. There are no psychiatrists or psychologists who occupy themselves with the personality of delinquents.

Infantile and Oligophrenic Psychiatry

Proceeding from a few observations, and above all through a comparison with other countries, Herbert Day Lamson in 1935 assumed that there were several million retarded in China. At that time, as today, studies of that question were extremely few. In 1930, Dr. A. H. Woods affirmed that "all degrees of oligophrenia are frequent in China."* In a study made in Peking in 1929 of forty minors in a reformatory, Yeng Ching-yueh demonstrated through the Binet Simon test, adapted for China, that four-fifths had an intelligence quotient of less than seventy.[32] Previously, the retarded were much more numerous because of privations of every type: undernourishment, infectious diseases like syphilis which cause hereditary changes, the lack of care before, during, and after delivery, and abandonment because of lack of means.

At the present time we do not know of any institution for the retarded. In the entire country there is only one service for child psychiatry. It has a twenty-four bed endowment and is located in the Psychiatric Hospital of Nanking, where I saw three schizophrenics treated with insulin. Denis Lazure of the Psychiatric Service of the Montreal Medical School states that one child-psychiatry unit inaugurated in a

* Chinese Medical Journal, 40:T 1070.

new psychiatric hospital in Shanghai had to be closed and transformed into a pavilion for adults, because during two years of operation only eight children were admitted. In Greater Shanghai until the end of 1957 there existed only one reformatory for delinquent minors. It held 121 boys and girls between thirteen and eighteen years of age, 90 percent of them for robberies and thefts. The director, who was not specially qualified in the subject, did not recognize among them the existence of mental deficients; in fact, deficients seemed to him more intelligent than average children.

The present attitude toward the retarded is to incorporate them in everyday life and work. Whereas the oligophrenics are cared for in their homes, the retarded, according to the educators' concept, do not require special classes inasmuch as the teachers and their more gifted companions dedicate much attention to them (Denis Lazure).

My impression is that the Chinese cultural norms resemble in this respect those of the societies of the South Seas natives which were studied by Margaret Mead. They make no distinction between the underendowed and the normal and avoid displays of superiority by the latter or by those who are overendowed; they accept the former such as they are, and they are accommodated to the culture insofar as possible. These attitudes in China reflect pedagogic inclination, since oligophrenia receives rather limited medical attention. The kindergartens and homes, the clubs and day nurseries, and the children's sections of unions and other large institutions give evidence of the care with which children, normal or abnormal, are surrounded.

Neuroses

The neuroses are not as widespread in China as they are in the West, and they are considered social rather than psychiatric problems, correctable through education or other means, as long as they do not have a frankly pathological character.

The majority of neuroses are classified as neurasthenia, which includes many symptoms: abnormal fatigue, anxiety, phobia, headaches, vexation, etc. In the 1959 symposium, Lo Ch'ung-p'ei and collaborators emphasized that psychasthenia was found in 60 percent of those treated by the mobile units of the Department of Mental Health, Peking College of Medicine, as well as in many other patients of various clinical and neurological departments. During the first half of 1959, the Faculty of Medicine of Peking made a study of 25,471 persons in the city, one people's commune, two lyceums, two faculties, three groups of artists, one state ware-house, and three district people's committees. It was found that 90.2 percent of the ill were between 16 and 40 years old. White-collar workers made up 54.4 percent of the population examined and manual workers 45.6 percent; 87.7 percent of the ill belonged to the first group and 13.3 percent to the second. Of those doing heavy manual labor, 68.7 percent showed signs of disease, whereas among those doing light work, the figure was 31.3 percent; however in the population studied, 86.4 percent performed light work and only 13.6 percent heavy work. The relation-ship between heavy, light, and white-collar work was 1:19:25. With medical students, the ratio between those taking basic courses and those who practiced was 2:1 or 3:1; of all those who contracted psychasthenia after entering medical school, 88.2 percent were in the basic courses. For those in high school, the frequency was similar for students in the first, second and third year of senior high school, with those in the third year most susceptible; the population ratio of third-year to first-year and second-year students combined was 4:9.

A curious syndrome of acute and transient anxiety, with a partial de-personalization syndrome which leads to the conviction of penis shrink-age and the fear of disintegration, has been described in Southeast China (Canton zone) under the name Suk-yeong, or Koro. It has also been found in Malaysia, Indonesia, and the South Celebes, and occasionally so has its equivalent among women, who complain of the shrinkage of the vulvar labia and breasts (Von Wulftfen Palthe). The most complete study is that of P. M. Yap,[31] who in more than fifteen years discovered nineteen cases in men in Hong Kong with immature personality, who varied in age from sixteen to forty-five years, who, with the exception of a bookkeeper, all belonged to the working class, and who all disclosed sexual histories plagued with conflicts and inhibitions. This is a syndrome whose form and content are determined by a combination of social and cultural factors acting on predisposed personalities. They responded to adequate psychotherapy, to tranquilizers, and, in extreme cases, to treat-ment with insulin and convulsive agents.

Delinquency and Imprisonment

Before the Liberation, Shanghai was reputed throughout the world for its criminality and drug traffic and for being the whorehouse of the Orient, the paradise of adventurers and gangsters. We interviewed, at the end of 1957, the President of the People's High Court and professor of one of the law faculties, Dr. Hen Sha-chin. Shanghai previously had numerous types of delinquency (he enumerated some thirty). The most frequent were robberies, highway robberies, corruption, abduction of persons, and sale of opium and other drugs. In hotels and buses the following small posters were always seen: "Beware of Pickpockets" or "Mind Your Own Clothing." According to the 1947 Yearbook, in 1946 there were 886 highway robberies, 510 murders, 10,446 robberies, and 8,168 cases of narcotics sales. There were opium and heroin dens at many street corners, and it is calculated that 1 out of every 80 families sold drugs. The cases of corruption were very numerous, but very few trials reached the courts for the reason that many functionaries of the Kuomintang government were accomplices and conspired to prevent these cases from coming to trial. The confidants and secret agents of the Kuomintang worked in complicity with the thieves, and consequently the important ones could not be arrested but only those of lesser account. It was characteristic of the courts that there were more penal than civil actions: In 1946 the penal cases totaled 71 percent.

After 1949, things began to change. Abductions of persons, the drug traffic, and forging of currency and documents ceased completely. The ratio of criminal to civil trials was changed: in 1950, 34.8 percent; in 1953, 26 percent; in 1956, 21.8 percent. Taking 1950 as a base, in 1956 the crime rate fell to only 17.7 percent. The decrease occurred particularly after 1955 because the socialist transformation of the urban and rural areas had been accentuated. Some forms of crime persisted, for example thefts and robberies, particularly in some branches of industry which were not well organized. In the beginning, the government took pains to arrest professional thieves, who in the most serious cases were condemned to death and otherwise to prolonged imprisonment. The problem was originally very grave because numerous police functionaries were accomplices of the thieves and of other types of delinquents.

Today, 90 percent of the personal-quarrel cases and personal-injury cases are resolved through intervention, arbitration, and critique. These minor cases are caused above all by inadequate living conditions and by hoarding; in contrast, quarrels between vagabonds or other persons in the streets, which previously were frequent, are the exception today. Only 10 percent of the quarrels result in prison sentences or fines.

The people's mobilization has contributed much to the reduction of delinquency, and even to its prevention. Previously individual life was

tolerated, and it was not known in one house what went on in the
neighboring house; now, neighbors know each other and communicate.
There is a very active social life; the conscience of the masses is being
formed. I was told of the case of a bank employee who stole 10,000 yens;
the next day his family denounced him. There are always those who do
not understand how it is possible to accuse one's own; it is that today
there is a new morality. The sanctions are more benign than formerly for
the one who transgresses only occasionally. For the one who has performed an antisocial act, an effort at reform is part of the punishment. The
principal cause for the reduction of delinquency is that the government
is built on the masses, and these help the government in every manner
and demonstrate year after year how they benefit in their material and
moral well-being.

In 1965 we visited the Municipal Prison of Peking, which houses
1,800 prisoners, divided into two groups: common delinquents, 60 percent;
counterrevolutionaries, 40 percent. Of the total, 100 are women. The
authorities informed me that the most frequent forms of delinquency are
robbery, fraud, and corruption of functionaries; homicides, assault, and
rape are very rare. The vast jail has seven wards, each of which has many
cells with two large sleeping platforms, each for four persons. The construction is ancient, but there is order and cleanliness. There are no longer
bars at the windows nor locks on the doors and the jailers and guards do
not carry arms. The staff consists of 120, including thirty on hospital
service and another thirty as security guards. The conveniences—ample
courtyards, a library, a shop, and many other social services—are excellent.
The hospital has fifty beds, and the director informs me that the majority
of those for whom it cares suffer from heart, stomach, and other physical
diseases. Cases of insanity, neurosis, or psychosomatic illnesses are exceptional; he believes that this is because the inmates see ample possibilities
for rehabilitation in the future.

Everybody works; one hundred percent of the jail population is
employed in two immense factories, one of which produces hosiery and
the other plastics of all types. Prisoners work eight hours per day, study
two, and have one hour for sports and diversions. They have theatrical
companies, a daily newspaper, movies, and other recreations; they are
taken to exhibits and invite outstanding workers from other factories,
with whom they hold conferences or give information about their methods
of work. The principle of reform is work and political education. The
following are a few steps in this process of reform: (a) a confession of

the crime and understanding of the damage which has been done to society and the State is expected; (b) a critique is rendered of their concepts, illusions, and reactionary ideas, giving evidence that these concepts are being rooted out as the socialists are triumphing; (c) the idea that work is the source of life and dignity is expounded and the tendency to scorn work and the techniques and abilities to interrupt work are criticized; (d) cultural and technical education in all forms is stimulated through competition and superior production is rewarded. Every month meetings and discussions are organized, and prizes, some 80 percent in money, are awarded. The prizes may also consist of a reduction in the sentence, and even of conditional liberty at the suggestion of the prison authorities (first the security department and then the courts). Punishments consist of warnings, dialogues about errors committed, and finally, an increase in the jail sentence. The immense majority enjoy rewards, and punishments are very rare. Criminological studies are the exception, and there is little preoccupation with the criminal pathological personality. It is felt that social causes of crime predominate and that in some prisoners a bourgeois ideology and the bad habits of earlier times still subsist.

The rehabilitation methods in the Wu Haa jail, according to what Raimando Fares relates, are similar to the ones described. The ratio of political to common criminals is greater: of 1,132 prisoners, 713 were political. That of the sexes is also different: 851 were men, 781 women.

Prostitution

According to the widely held but very controversial Lombroso theory, prostitution is the feminine equivalent to masculine delinquency. Shanghai was also the largest center of Chinese prostitution; it was one of the most flourishing businesses and one in which the functionaries participated. In 1925, 3,744 licenses were issued for the opening of houses of prostitution; in 1929 these licenses had increased to 8,767. "A large proportion of the creatures," Hauser reports, "came from Hanchu and Sochu, where they had been acquired for little money at their most tender age. In the regions exposed to floods and hunger, the purchasers could obtain them for a mouthful of bread. At the age of 13, these little girls spent their first night with one of the favored clients of the houses of tolerance."

It is calculated that during the first days of the Liberation there were 800 houses of prostitution, with 4,000 registered women, and more than 20,000 clandestine prostitutes. From 1949 to 1951, the People's Government concentrated its attention on consolidating and reforming the situation. It declared the public houses illegal and encouraged the prostitutes to return to their homes. Some of the women found honest work. Each time the political conscience of the population became aroused the mass organizations demanded the abolition of prostitution. In 1951, the People's Assembly of Shanghai promulgated the complete abolition. The government closed the seventy-two houses which still existed and adopted measures against the *souteneurs;* it detained those who were guilty of capital offenses or other crimes and treated with clemency those who deserved it, encouraging them to seek work.

Still, prostitution could not be abolished merely by decree; it was necessary also to change the women, not simply through coercion, but by promoting in them a state of conscience relative to the new social order. The great majority accepted the explanation and the education and through them caught a glimpse of a pleasant future in a new way of life. There were women who needed more time for their reform; there still remained a small proportion, less than 10 percent, of women of loose conduct and habits. The public-safety units then forced them to accept reform, to which end political education and work were used simultaneously. The content of the political education consisted of: (a) awakening their sensitivity toward self-respect and honor; (b) the observance of law and regulations; (c) promulgation of the idea that work is a matter of honor and it is shameful to live off the traffic of one's body; (d) culture classes, above all reading classes (for the majority were illiterate).

In the education centers, or reformatories, the functionaries gained the confidence of the internees at public gatherings, and later they conversed with them individually. At the same time they cured their venereal diseases, which affected some 70 percent, and other diseases, showing through photographs and by other means the damage these diseases caused. The patients attended classes for four hours and devoted four hours to work. The working hours could be increased, depending on the state of health and aptitude of the individual. Those who progressed more rapidly helped the others; through collective living, they gradually abandoned their tendency toward licentiousness. The wards enjoyed civil rights and quite a few liberties, but patients had to ask permission to leave. Upon discharge, they were helped in finding adequate work, and their origins were given consideration in this task. Seventy percent returned to their native countryside and agricultural cooperatives, where they could live from their work without necessity of owning land. Some twenty percent stayed in Shanghai or in other cities and gained employment in light industries, as nursemaids, or at domestic labor. The majority of the former wards formed new houses and acquired complete self-respect. It was very important that they should acquire the security of their substance. The ones who relapsed were rare, barely three per thousand. Not even in the reformatories were women with mental aberrations encountered; if they had them, they were attributed to the abjection and oppression under which they had lived.

The new cases of clandestine prostitution are scarce, but for those, reformatories are not needed; public education is sufficient; the neighbors and the district organizations help in preventing their recurrence. On the other hand, the degree of popular conscience has become such that the demand for prostitution practically does not exist.

Claude Roy eloquently explained what reform involves, the Chinese system being so far removed from what is done in other places. Former prostitutes, criminals, counterfeiters or spies, and minors with antisocial reactions, are organized in small groups of ten or twelve and an attempt is made to create a conscience in each of them. They are encouraged to public confession; and through intimate reform, in which all help and support one another, the footstep of each one is made to coincide with the rhythm of the footsteps of all. "If we use our personality for others and in the others and through the others, if the human being is characterized by what he gives to his fellow, and not by that which separates him from all, if man, instead of being a wolf toward man, is simply and at the same time his kind and his brother, his witness and his kin, then the People's China is right in counting upon the possibility that people are perfecting themselves and helping each other."

TRAINING OF PSYCHIATRIC PERSONNEL, TEACHING, AND DOCTRINES

In 1949, psychiatry was taught in most of the twenty-seven or thirty-eight (depending upon the authors) Chinese medical schools then in existence.

At present, psychiatry is taught in ninety medical schools, nineteen of which are traditional medical schools. Psychiatry is the fourth year of a six-year course of study. In 1957, in Peking, it was taught in an ancient, inadequate edifice which had been a private sanitarium, and which could lodge sixty patients. Plans called for it to be enlarged to 200 beds; however, by 1965, this had not yet been done.

The Chinese Medical College, founded in 1957, is a type of high-level medical faculty with an eight-year plan of study which stresses the basic subjects (mathematics, and the biological, physical, and chemical sciences). Every year, on the basis of examinations that test knowledge, ability, health, and political convictions, sixty students are allowed to enter. At least thirty must be from the proletarian class. Some of the professors were trained at the old Peking Union Medical College, others are graduates of the Chinese Medical College itself. The school has fourteen medical departments, of which two are for prophylactic medicine and two are clinical departments. In all fourteen, however, investigatory work is pursued. The lecture year is divided into thirty-eight weeks of study, six of manual labor, and eight of vacation. First-year students do the farm work; the ones in the upper classes work in the factories. Psychiatry is taught in the seventh year, and eighteen hours a week are devoted to seminars, forty to practical labors. Since the College does not have psychiatric beds, instruction is given in hospitals for the specialty. When I commented to Dr. Chang, the dean, an energetic and capable woman some sixty years old, on the scant attention which the school devoted to the teaching of psychiatry and medical psychology in comparison to other medical schools of the Orient and the Occident, she answered that the training in these matters was in the province of political education and etiquette, rather than of medicine.

At the Shanghai Psychiatric Institute, established in 1958, instruction is given in the fourth year to some 10,000 students assigned to two medical schools and the Railroad Hospital. Four groups of teachers have devoted themselves, respectively, to teaching, treatment, prophylaxis, and study.

Until the advent of Nazism, there were Chinese psychiatrists trained in Germany, and these generally had a predominantly Kraepelinian orientation. From 1933 on, students of psychiatry preferred to attend North American schools, and many developed psychoanalytical orientations. Since 1949, the influence of Pavlovian doctors has been very dominant. The textbook by Gilyarowsky—dominant in Soviet psychiatry—has been translated into Chinese and is used in medical schools. Soviet psychiatrists gave courses at the medical faculties, and centers for the study of the higher nervous system were established. Since the estrangement from the U.S.S.R., Chinese psychiatrists are taking pains to elaborate a psychiatry with a national mark, without having this national isolationism exclude knowledge of contributions being made in the different schools of the world.

We have not encountered any book or article in which the prevailing doctrine in present Chinese psychiatry is clearly expressed. Throughout the works in progress and from conversations with the most objective psychiatrists, it seems to me that they are oriented along two principal lines. In the first place, they are concerned with the exceedingly important role of the social, ecological, and environmental factors in the etiology and development of psychoses and neuroses (not to infer disregard of the endogenic, constitutional, and dispositional causes or of the clinics themselves). On the other hand, after having followed, with extreme Chinese faithfulness and tenacity, the teachings of various schools, and especially that of Pavlov in its penultimate stage, they are presently on the way toward elaborating their own concept. Without neglecting the characteristics of the individual personality, the tendency is to understand psychiatric infirmities on the basis of the organic-psychic unity. Scientific interchange, after the estrangement from the Soviet Union and a bloc of other nations, is reduced to a minimum. Even though Chinese psychiatrists follow with interest the international scientific movement through the publications, they rarely attend congresses on the outside. They tend to make their own experience in a world for themselves. Their investigations are centered on the clinical, electroencephalographic, biochemical, neurophysical, and therapeutic aspects. At the present time, it appears that there do not exist any studies under way on comparative and transcultural psychiatry or on the relationships between psychopathological syndromes and social, ethnic, and cultural conditioning. The ways of traditional medicine are being abandoned—even though they are trying to salvage that which is truly useful in it—in order to continue with Western science. After so many centuries of ignorance and deviation, they are rapidly raising their standards of methodology and practice, with characteristic intelligence and tenacity. They have a long, a very long way to walk, but they have entered this path resolutely.

A RATIONAL DIRECTIVE PSYCHOTHERAPY

Although psychotherapy does not exist as a specialty in China, it is nevertheless being practiced. Frequently physicians and psychiatrists will regard human problems as amenable to treatment either by themselves or by health workers, nurses, relatives, or friends, and particularly by the political educator. The Chinese are certainly far from ignoring these problems and have attempted to create a psychotherapeutic doctrine. Though they do not acknowledge the prevailing Western doctrines which, since

Freud, have stressed the exploration of the unconscious, they have developed their own practical methods. It is well known that they repudiate psychoanalysis and the various schools that have been derived from it. For a time they adopted Pavlovian interpretations: conditioning, reconditioning, the strengthening or weakening of inhibition, and stimulation of weak points. They still do take these processes into consideration, however, at present, they are not essential in practice.

Chinese psychotherapy goes its own way, and although no coherent body of principles has as yet been elaborated, the main outlines may be perceived. They constitute a rational directive psychotherapy which incorporates forces of conscience, the call for an individual effort, and engagement by education and reeducation within the framework of the current sociopolitical conditions and the prevailing political thinking, dialectic materialism.

The neurotic is no passive witness to his illness or suffering, not the object of medical treatment by means of medication, psychotherapeutic or physiotherapeutic methods; he must fight the disease and its symptoms. At the start of the treatment, the psychiatrist begins by explaining to the patient the origin, nature, and course of his illness, the negative and troublesome traits of his personality, and the treatment he is to undergo. The rare predilection for applying suggestion or hypnotherapy is thus easy to understand. Another characteristic of Chinese psychotherapy is the participation of the group in the individual's recovery, the interest the others take in helping him, and the principle that "the strong must help the weak." In factories, in offices, in the country, in the communes—everywhere—his superiors and companions collaborate in a significant effort to make the patient feel good; instead of isolating him, ridiculing his strange symptoms, separating him, or setting him apart, they take an active interest in him and encourage his recovery. The political doctrine is not only a theory of government but is also the practice of human and social solidarity.

For a better understanding of how this psychotherapy is practiced, we shall report on procedures in two groups of patients, the first suffering from psychasthenia, an entity grouped among the neurasthenias and other neurotic conditions, the second consisting of chronic psychotics.

The method of treatment in psychasthenia combines physiotherapy and psychotherapy and requires approximately one month. The former consists of various medications (Pavlov's mixture of caffeine and bromide [for which a psychopharmacologic drug may be substituted, preferably

Ampliactil], insulin in small doses, Chinese herbs, hormones, nerve tonics, and stimulants), novocain, electric sleep (progressively diminishing), physical and respiratory exercises, and iron therapy. The psychotherapeutic treatment is a combination of individual and group therapy on a nonanalytical basis. It comprises three principles or basic elements:

1. Help the patient understand his illness fully, call on his sense of responsibility, and imbue him with optimism for a rapid recovery. Strive to keep him attentive and alert, disperse his fears and worries, and increase his confidence in the possibility of recovery. It is felt that the sense of responsibility to his country and to socialism constitutes an unlimited source of energizing power.

2. Let the patient know about his illness. Its origin, development, deterioration, and recovery follow an objective, regular pattern. Once the patient understands this pattern he can more easily adopt an active attitude. Instead of passively accepting his illness he himself may push toward recovery.

3. Try to stimulate development of the patient's own subjective activity; the authors call this "active subjectivity and creativity" in the struggle against the disease. Efforts are made toward having the patient relate the objective pattern of his disease to the specific conditions of his environment and his own personality so as to formulate a practical approach for combating the illness and its symptoms. This is a long-term proposition; it includes judicious, rather methodical organization of work and study and a sensible, ordered life. It also includes recreation, cultural activities, and physical exercise. The patient should try to correct his bad temperamental traits.

In a clinic with 1,042 ambulatory patients where combined treatment was given for three to five weeks, 80 percent were much improved; a three months' follow-up showed that the improvement had been maintained in 78 percent of the cases. The results were attributed to social consciousness and to the fact that every patient had the impetus to act and struggle against the disease (i.e., to respond to the psychotherapy). Detailed explanation and elucidation addressed to the patient is considered essential in the latter.[4] In a recent survey on 1,160 patients, a new therapeutic plan divided into three stages was announced: (a) During the first three to five days mutual understanding is established between patient, physician, and environment; (b) Treatment is offered to relieve primary and secondary symptoms; (c) Consolidation of treatment in combination with physical and mental exercises is offered. These are designed to prepare the patient for his return to work after he is discharged. There were 15.26 percent recoveries, 61.88 percent near recoveries, and 19.2 percent improvements.

In the case of the hospitalized patients, we have seen that physicians and the rest of the personnel strove to establish good contact with them because this opens the path for careful individual treatment. Collective cultural and physical activities are organized (choirs, dances, parties, rhythmical exercises, outings) which enrich the patients' lives. To draw them out of their isolation and away from the symptoms and anxieties to which they cling, their interest in everyday events and political happenings is aroused. To this effect, reunions and meetings are organized where these issues are discussed. This could be considered as collective therapy (of a frequently political nature) rather than as group psychotherapy. Naturally work therapy also exists, but we have as yet seen no compact system developed by the Chinese psychiatrists.

The emphasis on education, reeducation and rehabilitation of neurotics might be hard for the Western mind to understand unless we considered the characteristics of the Revolution in China and the history of their thinking, which is realistic and practical, avoiding formal investigations and speculations without a concrete basis. The system differs from methods of education and reeducation such as those explained by Pierre Janet.*

In a related field, Claude Roy points out that the methods for rehabilitating delinquents, abandoned minors, former prostitutes, spies, and forgers are fundamentally the same. In place of punishment or moralizing sermons, an attempt is made to create in these individuals a moral and social conscience. This is frequently initiated with a public confession. Internal reform is conceived as an undertaking in which all help and support each other: The search for truth and the conquest of liberty cannot be achieved by the individual; it requires the efforts of organized groups.† If we hold our personality by virtue of the others, in the others, and through the others, comments Roy, "If a human being is characterized by what he gives to his fellow-creature rather than by what separates him from all the others, if man, instead of prying on man, could be simply both his mirror and his brother, his witness and his *alter ego;*

---

* Described in the second volume of *Medications Psychologiques*, Paris, 1919.
† In the publication of the French Dominican Order, *La Vie intellectuelle*, it is pointed out that this is a very old truth of the Church: "A Catholic should be the last to show surprise or indignation at this organization of collectives, since he professes and lives in his faith only by the Church."

then the Chinese people are definitely right in counting with the possibility that human beings can mutually perfect and help each other."

The author adds that what defines China as distinct from the Occident is their different notions of discretion and private life. The attitude of members of one community toward another in the former appears as a sort of objective and tolerant benevolence rather than envy or hostility; the human being is an object of interest rather than one of apprehension. This quite general feeling of living under everybody's eyes has for centuries been linked to a no less general feeling of being responsible for all the others. Man's solidarity with society is extended to include all of nature. "Criticism and self-criticism in China are not more than a concretion of an ancient certainty: that of the oneness of humanity, that of harmony between the colors of the souls and the sound of the spirits; that of an existing mysterious and evident interrelationship between man, the universe, and society."

This conviction, he says, has been expressed by the Fathers of the Church when they conceived the Dogma of the Communions of Saints, by Marx when he said that in communism "human brotherhood is not a phrase, it is a reality," and by other thinkers, philosophers, and reformers. The transformation achieved has been eloquently expressed by a member of an organized gang which had engaged in robbery, illicit traffic, and mugging. He said: "Before, the question in my gang was, who would do more *against* the people; now it is, who would do more *for* the people."

PSYCHOTHERAPY OF CHRONIC PSYCHOTICS IN THE SHANGHAI CONVALESCENT HOME

I had visited several psychiatric hospitals in Shanghai but wanted to get acquainted with other evidence of the specialists' activities; I therefore asked Professor Hsuh Tsung-hwa, director of the main mental hospital of the city, to show me another, different institution, and he took me to the Convalescent Home.

The Convalescent Home is located in the Shanghai outskirts. It consists of several old dilapidated houses which previously had constituted a private sanitarium; the administration was about a hundred meters from the central building. When reform of operations of these private sanitariums was instituted by the State in 1956, its owner transferred it voluntarily to the State and continued to work there. In 1958, it was renamed the Convalescent Home, and the operative reform began in 1960, using the new methods described below.

It housed about fifty-five women who entered it in a state of severe chronic dementia, all of whom had a history of from four to fifteen years illness; all had been in other mental hospitals. When they arrived, they were disheveled, dirty, incapable of personal care, and in a state of deep mental and frequently also physical prostration.

The treatment was divided into four stages:

1. To start these human residues moving, these remains with hardly a mental glimmer, to rescue them from their deep autism, it was decided to begin with one of the most deep-rooted vital elements, rhythm. They were thus first given music therapy. The patients were divided into groups of ten to twelve led by assistants. They heard music every day for one to two hours. This was not just any music; it consisted essentially of stimulating, exciting songs, full of vitality and capable of arousing enthusiasm, revolutionary songs in particular. In the beginning the patients did not seem interested, but it did not matter whether or not they responded to the music. Most, if not all, started to react after ten to twenty days; they followed the songs with their hands and feet, gestured, and accompanied the music with head movements. This was continued for a month and a half to two months until the patients sang the songs themselves. I myself was impressed to see these patients, earlier so demented, sing about ten songs in my presence. Three to four months passed in this way to verify whether there was true improvement corresponding to the degree in which they cooperated in these music sessions. At the end of that stag, they started to participate in group activities, always under the direction of an aide.

2. Now they had to acquire new habits; this was the rehabilitation which is part of any therapy for chronic cases. It required patience from the physician, nurse, or group leader, infinite, as that of a mother for her child. The patients got up at six o'clock in the morning, washed, took care of their personal hygiene, brushed their teeth, made their beds, and straightened their rooms. In the beginning they were taken by the hand and shown step by step how to perform these activities. After a time, both the patients and their surroundings, earlier so deteriorated and dirty, adopted norms of cleanliness and became orderly. For main meals or breakfast they stood in line and were taught how to eat and what manners to adopt.

In the beginning, twenty-five persons had been required for the care of forty patients. Now only six nurses were needed for fifty-five patients.

3. The third stage aimed at restoring intelligence. The patients had forgotten almost everything and now had to be shown things and acts in every detail. At the start, one person told stories and encouraged responses and conversation. The patients were taken to exhibitions and for walks. Their interest in other activities of daily life was stimulated. Four times a week there were sessions using TV, radio, movies, and readings from journals and magazines. When their condition permitted, they attended classes one or several times weekly to learn arithmetic, their Chinese idiom, and other subjects. Then they were taught mental hygiene. They listened to talks on the meaning of mental disease, were told that this is not a disgrace, and were taught ways to get rid of their illness.

At this stage, the patients began to take note of each other, and learned to organize their daily lives. They were encouraged to write about their own experiences and to report their impressions. Sometimes self-education is more effective than that offered by the physicians. This stage takes three or four months.

4. When the patients were able to occupy themselves, relationship with their families and environment was reestablished. The patients were permitted to go home on visits for one to three days. It was then determined whether their condition was such as to enable them to stay with their families. If such was the case, they were discharged from the hospital. However, the nurse always visited their homes every two days and then every four, five, or more days. In the meantime, the social worker who had visited the family gave them instructions and suggestions on their life, study, and work.

These four periods together usually take one year. For patients in a favorable state, about six months will be sufficient. About 80 percent of the patients recover or show considerable improvement. They are at least not destructive, aggressive, or dirty, and they can take care of themselves. About 10 to 15 percent are released after six months; they usually return to the work they did before. No change is seen in 10 to 15 percent of the cases.

Prior to entering the Home, these patients had been subjected to highly diverse therapies: insulin shock, electroshock, and neuroleptics. During the course of reeducation they occasionally had to take neuroleptics, hynotics, or other medication, usually up to 150 mg. chlorphromzine or at most 200 mg.

Professor Hsuh told me that he began to think about the possibility of applying this method after reading Mao's work *On Contradiction*. Each thing in the world has its opposite. If the patient has features of abnormality he must have other features of normality. The patient himself is a contradiction. Those features may be exchanged, one against the other. Mental patients suffer greatly in their innermost self. They feel despised, they live in isolation. Accordingly, the first and foremost treatment is that physician and hospital personnel be the patients' friends and show them their sympathy. They must share their lives at meals, work, and recreation and even sleep nearby. This is done by the staff in the required degree. The patients must be restored to life, and therefore, they must be accompanied without uniforms, without white aprons, without the exercise of rigid authority.

The budget is very low. The cost for each patient amounts to 2 yens per day, thus less than a dollar.

The point of departure of the treatment is music and songs. Since antiquity, the value of music therapy in neuroses and psychoses has been known. In this sense there exists a millennial tradition in China which may be traced back as far as Confucius. His sixth book is the *Book of Music,* entered in Lin-Yu-Tang's work, *The Wisdom of Confucius,* which is mentioned by Rolf Krojanker:

When the chord of the heart is touched by pain the sounds produced are somber and solitary; when the chord of the heart is touched by satisfaction, the sounds will be languid and slow; those of happiness, bright and expansive; those of anger, harsh and strong; those of compassion, simple and pure; those of love, sweet and gentle. These six forms of emotion are not spontaneous, they are produced by the impact of the external world . . . The kings of antiquity gave much attention to what affects the human heart . . . The ancient kings did not institute rites and music with the exclusive aim of satisfying the desire of our senses, but rather to teach the people correct wisdom and the return to normality.

Music and songs are important, but they are not the sole treatment and sometimes not even its most important part. The physicians' and staff's devotion play a great role. Nothing is more important in the therapy of neurotics or psychotics than the therapist himself, the human element, the warm solidarity shown in attending to the patients. The importance of participation by physician and personnel and the extent to which their devotion contributes toward pulling the patients out of the pit into which they have progressively been sinking, should be elucidated and defined. Their attention may occasionally be compared to that of a mother for her child or a teacher for the very young. In the Convalescent Home, nurses and even the physician, if necessary, will share their patients' lives, eat with them, sleep close by, without uniform, without rigid rules. We should also stress the importance of this kind of therapy in groups. It is the group which helps the individual, supports him, stimulates him, and urges him on. This is not exactly group psychotherapy as it is usually understood. The fact that the Chinese, more than other people, have participated for thousands of years in the group life of the family and of work, on the communal, municipal and national levels renders them more sensitive to this type of collective, group psychotherapy. Here, as on other occasions, psychotherapy must pay attention to the traditional sociocultural values of each people.

A Gigantic Communal Movement for Mental Health

The newest projects in the mental health movement are the community centers for mental health.* Their concept derives from the realization that the classic programs of mental hygiene were useless or thoroughly insufficient, as was the idea that mobilizing the psychiatrists would in some way lead to program promotion. For such goals, active and conscious participation by various sectors of the population is indispensable, both in the planning and in the execution of the developmental programs at the different communal levels: local, regional, and national. More than an economic impulse is required for the development and well-being of the people; psychological forces must be stimulated and obstacles which have been accumulated by routine, inveterate habits, and the systems of traditional values must be removed. Among definitions for the mobilization of communities, the following has been proposed: "Community organization is a type of social service referring to all efforts tending to efficiently direct social resources towards meeting the specific or total needs of a delimited area. Their tasks may include activities such as searching for data, developing plans for social welfare, changes of systems or patterns of social services or for the promotion of social legislation."

Such a plan was a particular necessity for the Chinese people. Their miseries and their physical and moral suffering were so oppressive and of

* See *International Trends in Mental Health,* ed. Henry P. David, McGraw-Hill Book Company Series in International Development, 1965. The main parameters of the *Community Mental Health Journal* are: programming of services for prevention and control of mental changes, planning for community organization, studies of psychiatric epidemiology, and many other tasks.

such colossal magnitude that only a social earthquake like the Revolution could set them on the road toward achieving satisfactory mental health. The Revolution smashed individualism, promoted solidarity, and mobilized the people's resources in a constant of activity in the new conditions of collective living.

It is amazing that such significant results could have been obtained in so little time and in such an immense country, the most populated in the world, and one loaded down with tradition. By forcing our imagination, we might be able to envision the colossal resources and forces needed to effect results similar to those obtained there if Occidental norms of mental hygiene had been put into practice, with their network in institutions, psychiatrists, social workers, psychologists, health officers, etc. Though it is absurd to think that such could have been made available, if so, they would probably not have given satisfactory results under the present living conditions, for reasons too complex to explain. Furthermore, had the earlier conditions persisted, under which a large part of the population were living in hovels, lacking elementary hygiene, undernourished, weakened by opium and alcohol and exhausted by long hours of work, the Chinese would have continued endlessly to produce new multitudes of sick and abnormal creatures. There is no doubt that the road to mental health must pass through that of well-being.

Effective and simple methods are necessary to meet the needs, mentality, and customs of the masses of an immense nation. These are the master lines of well-being, which is attained by hard toil and austere discipline. It is achieved, not through liberty as it is understood in the Occident, but through a creative freedom which may be as ample as desired if practiced within the framework of national objectives. After facing the exploitation of the great majority of the population, the resulting chaos, the terrible war of invasion and the civil war, the hypocritical violence of the rulers, the cynicism of a decadent morality, the Chinese people consider the present rule satisfactory and adequate with ample perspectives for the future.

Thus, problems of mental health are inextricably linked to and form part of the substance and process of national life and constitute some of the most basic political and humane concerns. Mental, moral, spiritual, and social health are intimately interwoven; they are inseparable. We can assert without exaggeration, therefore, that the Chinese revolutionary tempest proved an effective protagonist for the enthronement of mental health, for it swept away the corrupt remnants of a disintegrating society to impose new norms of living. The Revolution, however, is only the beginning of a great work and, like jewelers, its leaders and squadrons must persistently fashion the gold brought to light so as to make the human jewel shine in all its splendor. They certainly have a long way to go, for this endeavor is an unending road like life itself.

This is the principal lesson of the progress of mental health in China. If there is truth in Paul Sivadon's statement that in matters of mental health all countries are "on the road to development," China has jumped one or more difficult and costly stages by swiftly passing through custodial psychiatry and on to the therapeutic community. China today is a gigantic therapeutic community; its people and its government contribute actively to the solution of important health problems. Thanks to its revolution it has moved from a sociopathologic state directly to a state of social health.

References

1. BARNES AND BECKER: "Historia del Pensamiento Social," vol. I, Fondo de Cultura Economica, 1945.
2. JAN CERNY: Chinese Psychiatry, International Journal of Psychiatry, 1:2 (1965).
3. CHANG FENG-C'UN: Chinese Journal of Neurology and Psychiatry (1) 1958.
4. CHAO YI-CH-CH'ENG: Neurology, Neurosurgery and Psychiatry in New China, Chinese Medical Journal, 83:732 (1965).
5. BRUNO FRIEDMAN: Qu'y-a-t-il derrière la science chinoise? Science et vie, June, 1965.
6. F. G. HALPERN: "Notes on Medicine, including Neurology and Psychiatry," Chiu Yih Book Company, Shanghai.
7. W. HARTNER: Heilkunden in alten China, Sinica, 17 (1942).
8. J. L. HARVEY: Estimate of Insane in China, China Medical Journal, 34: 1920.
9. HSIA CHEN-YI: Chinese Journal of Neurology and Psychiatry, 4 (2):89 (1958).
10. HSU CH'ANG-LIN, YEN SHIH-YING, FU CHUNG-CHUN, CHANG POCHING, AND SU TSUNG-HWA: Therapeutic Effects of Roasted Rice and Flour Powder in the Termination of Insulin Shock, Chinese Journal of Neurology and Psychiatry, 3 (1) (1957).
11. E. H. HUME: "Doctors East, Doctors West: An American Physicians' Life in China," W. W. Norton & Company Incorporated, New York, 1946.
12. "International Trends in Mental Health," ed. Henry P. David, McGraw-Hill Book Company (Series in International Development), New York, 1965.
13. J. G. KERR: The "Refuge of the Insane" Canton, China Medical Missionary Journal, 12 (1898).
14. HERBERT DAY LAMSON: "Social Pathology in China," The Commercial Press, Shanghai, 1935.
15. LEE T'AO, CH'ENG CHIH-FAN, AND CHANG CH'I-SHAN: Some Early Records of Nervous and Mental Diseases in Traditional Chinese Medicine, Chinese Medical Journal, 81 (1962).
16. LEE T'AO: Chinese Medicine during the Chin and Yuan Eras, Chinese Medical Journal, 73 (1955).
17. ———: Chinese Medicine during the Ming Dynasty, Chinese Medical Journal, 76 (1958).
18. LI TEH-CHUAN: Health Work in New China, People's China, October 1, 1950.
19. R. S. LYMAN et al.: "Social and Psychological Studies in Neuropsychiatry in China," Division of Neuropsychiatry, Peking Union Medical College, Peking, 1939.

20. LIU SHAO-CHI: "How to Be A Good Communist," Foreign Languages Press, Peking, 1964.
21. J. L. MCCARTNEY: Neuropsychiatry in China: A Preliminary Observation, Chinese Medical Journal, 40 (1926).
22. ———: Neuropsychiatry in China: A Retrospect of Diagnosis, Chinese Medical Journal, 40 (1926).
23. E. A. POPOV: Zh. Nevropat. Psikhiat, 59 (10):1179 (1959).
24. POW MENG-YAP: International Journal of Psychiatry, 1 (2):246 (1965).
25. Program of Topics and Speakers for Session of May 19, 1938, Club Institute of the Shanghai Women's Associations, Shanghai, China.
26. Report of Committee In Psychiatry, Fourth Biennial Conference, Chinese Medical Association, 1937.
27. CHARLES HART WESTBROOK: Psychiatry and Mental Hygiene in Shanghai: Historical Sketch, The American Journal of Psychiatry, 110 (4) (1953).
28. K. C. WONG: A Short History of Psychiatry and Mental Hygiene in China, Chinese Medical Journal, 44 (1950).
29. K. C. WONG AND LIEN-TEH WU: "History of Chinese Medicine," Kellev and Walsh, Shanghai, 1920.
30. A. H. WOODS: The Incidence of Nervous Diseases in China, China Medical Journal, 40 (1926).
31. P. M. YAP: Koro—A Culture-bound Depersonalization Syndrome, British Journal of Psychiatry, 111:43–50 (1965).
32. YENG CHING-YEUH: "A Study on Crime in Peiping," Yenching University, 1929.

Epilogue

THIS VOLUME has been prepared with a number of objectives. Foremost has been the desire to include reports on all the Communist countries and to make these reports comprehensive enough to acquaint the Western world with the general trends in Communist psychiatry.

Some may argue that insofar as the authors' various ideological and national biases have encouraged distortions, their accounts are invalid. Such critics may feel that an unbiased foreign observer might have better assessed the trends, strengths, and weaknesses. I would answer that it is equally important to know what people think they are doing and what they wish to emphasize in their work. This volume includes chapters by representatives of the different Communist countries; despite a certain measure of expected uniformity, their reports are considerably varied.

Of particular interest is the varying extent to which Marxist-Leninist theory is interwoven with psychiatric theory and practice and even the results of treatment. It is difficult to determine the true significance of this ideological orientation in the psychiatry. Although there can be little doubt that it has greatly affected the organization of psychiatric care, it seems to have had less effect on theory, which remains essentially of an organic, physiological nature. Indeed, the emphasis on environmental factors seems quite compatible with more recent developments in the physiologically oriented schools.

As to the Soviet assertion that Communist social change has decreased the incidence and prevalence of psychiatric disorders, we must await further studies and a longer period of time to assess such a historical trend. In any event, data in the chapter on Yugoslavia point in a different direction, as does Gnat's recent work, which shows an increased incidence of disorders in a new settlement. Surely one should not minimize the contribution of such factors as war, migration, industrialization, and mechanization to differential morbidity rates.

Although we need more data to evaluate the efficacy of psychohygienic measures and psychoprophylaxis, there is little question that most Communist countries provide care for a wide segment of their populations whose mental health is recognized as an important ingredient of a successful society. As in any medical system founded on public health principles, emphasis is given to those forms of treatment which can be inexpensively, rapidly, and widely applied. This orientation seems consistent with the overall goals of the various regimes and, in recent years, with extensive use of the psychopharmaceutical agents which have so greatly changed the picture of mental illness throughout the world.

There can be little doubt that certain uniformities, especially in organization and theory, prevail in the Communist countries and that they have been influenced by Communist ideology. Many of the same trends, however, have occurred in non-Communist countries as well—for example, the development of nationalized mental services in the United Kingdom and in the Scandinavian countries and the persistence of Pavlovian research elsewhere. In this sense one can say that Communism per se, though undoubtedly crucial, may not have been the necessary precursor to the kinds of developments that have taken place in Communist countries.

It should be pointed out, too, that historical and cultural factors have contributed to significant differences between the Communist countries' psychiatries. Thus we should consider their war experiences, ethnic composition, extent of socialization or Communism, economic and social development, psychiatric traditions, and contact with developments in Western Europe. Events in the past decade—the gradual estrangement of China and the Eastern bloc, the emergence of nationalism in Rumania and other Eastern European countries, and the introduction of certain capitalistic economic measures in the Soviet Union—suggest that nationalist sentiments, grounded in various historical and cultural traditions, have more importance than is ordinarily attributed to them. Certainly the studies in this volume attest to the significance of nationalist traditions in psychiatry. Thus, while clinical research dominates Rumanian, Hungarian, and East German psychiatry, epidemiological studies have been especially developed in Poland, Czechoslovakia, Russia, and Bulgaria, and dynamically oriented psychotherapy currently flourishes in Yugoslavia.

The present survey leads us to conclude that Communist countries share the problems besetting psychiatry in the West. This is particularly true with regard to the psychoses, especially the schizophrenias, and to old age and adolescence, which are apparently the most problematic age groups in industrializing societies. The studies point, then, to problems, interests, goals, and purposes shared with psychiatrists elsewhere. It is hoped that a consideration of these common areas of concern will suggest direction for collaborative efforts. In fact, comparative studies may contribute the most to psychiatry by investigating the effects of environmental stress and social change on the incidence and prevalence of disorders.

Index